THE GLAUCOMA HANDBOOK

Glaucoma, the "silent thief of sight," is one of the leading causes of irreversible blindness. This engaging text unravels the complexities of this multifaceted condition. From the anatomy of the eye and mechanisms of disease to cutting-edge treatments and research, it bridges foundational knowledge with the latest advancements. Through case studies, patient narratives, and a focus on global disparities, it highlights the human impact of glaucoma and the importance of innovation and collaboration in combating it. It is a must-read for clinicians, researchers, and students seeking to deepen their understanding, improve patient outcomes, and explore the future of vision preservation.

Key Features

- Addresses a critical need for a comprehensive, multidisciplinary resource on glaucoma that bridges clinical practice, cutting-edge research, and global health perspectives
- Focuses on integrating clinical insights and emerging trends like AI, minimally invasive glaucoma surgeries (MIGS), and advanced imaging tools, making it a relevant resource for clinicians and researchers
- Includes patient narratives and real-world case studies, emphasizing the human side of glaucoma and fostering empathy and a deeper connection between practitioners and patients

THE GLAUCOMA HANDBOOK

Evidence-Based Clinical Care

Cansu Yüksel Elgin

CRC Press
Taylor & Francis Group
Boca Raton London New York

CRC Press is an imprint of the
Taylor & Francis Group, an **informa** business

Designed cover image: Cover image created by Ceyhun Elgin

First edition published 2026
by CRC Press
2385 NW Executive Center Drive, Suite 320, Boca Raton, FL 33431

and by CRC Press
4 Park Square, Milton Park, Abingdon, Oxon, OX14 4RN

CRC Press is an imprint of Taylor & Francis Group, LLC

ISBN: 978-1-041-08719-9 (hbk)
ISBN: 978-1-041-08721-2 (pbk)
ISBN: 978-1-003-64669-3 (ebk)

DOI: 10.1201/9781003646693

Typeset in Minion Pro
by Apex CoVantage, LLC

To my beloved daughter Akça and spouse Ceyhun Elgin

CONTENTS

PREFACE

Glaucoma stands as one of ophthalmology's most significant challenges, quietly robbing millions worldwide of their sight, often without noticeable symptoms until considerable vision loss has occurred. Despite advances in medical science and technology, glaucoma remains a leading cause of irreversible blindness globally, underscoring the urgent need for comprehensive, evidence-based strategies for its prevention, diagnosis, and management.

This book, *The Glaucoma Handbook: Evidence-Based Clinical Care*, arises from my ambition to bridge the persistent gap between rapidly advancing glaucoma science and real-world clinical practice. Glaucoma care is complex and continuously evolving, and thus clinicians, researchers, and policymakers alike require an authoritative resource that not only provides the latest scientific insights but also translates these insights into practical clinical guidance.

The genesis of this book lies in my recognition that, while abundant literature exists on glaucoma, much of it is fragmented, highly specialized, or inaccessible to general practitioners and healthcare providers operating outside tertiary care settings. My goal was clear from the outset: to create a unified, accessible, yet rigorous compendium of current knowledge and best practices that could meaningfully impact patient outcomes worldwide. Structured carefully to facilitate both comprehensive reading and quick reference, each chapter of this handbook systematically explores critical aspects of glaucoma care. Beginning with foundational concepts—including anatomy, physiology, and pathophysiology—the book progresses logically through clinical diagnosis; medical, surgical, and laser treatment modalities; and recent innovations. Special attention is paid to the challenges faced in pediatric populations, management of secondary glaucomas, and intersections with systemic diseases, reflecting the complexities practitioners encounter daily.

An emphasis on practical application permeates the text, demonstrated vividly through illustrative case studies, patient testimonials, and pragmatic discussions about patient adherence and cost-effective care strategies. Recognizing the profound influence of socioeconomic, cultural, and systemic barriers on patient care, this handbook also dedicates substantial discourse to public health dimensions, telemedicine, and culturally informed approaches to eye care, ensuring relevance across diverse global settings.

Moreover, the inclusive nature of this handbook—addressing clinicians, surgeons, public health professionals, researchers, and advocates—is aimed at fostering a multidisciplinary dialogue essential for transformative glaucoma care. Drawing from extensive professional experience and an awareness of both developed and resource-limited environments, I have sought to underscore the universal yet context-specific nature of glaucoma care. Ultimately, my ambition with the current book is not merely to inform but to inspire proactive change. I envision this book as a catalyst, equipping professionals to better serve their communities, empower their patients, and advocate effectively for greater global attention and resources to combat glaucoma. The journey toward improved glaucoma management and prevention is ongoing and demanding, yet profoundly rewarding. I invite readers to join me on this critical path toward preserving vision and enhancing the quality of life for millions worldwide.

AUTHOR

Dr. Cansu Yüksel Elgin is an Assistant Professor of Ophthalmology at Istanbul University–Cerrahpasa in Turkiye, with over a decade of clinical and research experience in glaucoma and anterior segment disorders. After earning her MD from Cerrahpasa Faculty of Medicine, she completed her ophthalmology residency at the same institution. She later pursued postdoctoral research at NYU Langone Medical Center, contributing to several high-impact projects on teleophthalmology, glaucoma progression, and AI in ophthalmic diagnostics.

Dr. Yüksel Elgin is a Fellow of both the European Board of Ophthalmology and the International Council of Ophthalmology. Her research interests span from surgical outcomes in trabeculectomy to the ethical and systemic implications of AI-driven ophthalmic care. She has authored numerous peer-reviewed publications and book chapters and maintains active memberships in the American Academy of Ophthalmology, the Turkish Ophthalmology Society, and the European Contact Lens Society.

CHAPTER 1
INTRODUCTION: UNDERSTANDING GLAUCOMA

Glaucoma remains a formidable global health challenge, silently affecting millions of individuals around the world and presenting an ongoing threat to vision and quality of life. Despite remarkable advances in diagnostic technologies and therapeutic interventions, glaucoma continues to pose substantial difficulties for healthcare providers, public health officials, and patients alike. This introductory chapter sets the foundation for understanding glaucoma not only as a clinical entity but as a complex issue intersecting with history, epidemiology, and healthcare delivery systems.

In the first section, "What Is Glaucoma? A Historical Perspective," we explore the historical trajectory of glaucoma, tracing how its definition, understanding, and treatments have evolved through the ages. By examining significant milestones—from ancient civilizations' initial descriptions to contemporary breakthroughs—we gain invaluable insights into the evolving nature of medical knowledge and practice. Following this historical context, the second section, "Epidemiology: Global Burden and Public Health Impact," addresses the extensive worldwide impact of glaucoma. Here, we analyze prevalence and incidence rates, exploring demographic and geographic variations. Highlighting public health implications, this section underscores the urgent need for targeted interventions, early detection, and accessible care strategies to mitigate glaucoma's global burden. Finally, in "Why This Book? Bridging the Gap between Science and Practice," the third section articulates the essential purpose of this handbook. This book seeks not only to synthesize the latest scientific evidence but to effectively translate it into actionable insights for everyday clinical practice. The ultimate objective is to empower practitioners and policymakers to improve patient outcomes through evidence-based strategies, fostering a global community committed to confronting and overcoming the challenges posed by glaucoma.

SECTION 1—WHAT IS GLAUCOMA? A HISTORICAL PERSPECTIVE

Glaucoma, one of the leading causes of irreversible blindness globally, possesses a rich history that spans several millennia. This historical narrative not only highlights significant advancements in medical understanding and practice but also illustrates persistent challenges faced in the management and comprehension of this complex disease.

DOI: 10.1201/9781003646693-1

The term "glaucoma" derives from the ancient Greek word "glaukos," signifying a bluish-green coloration observed in affected eyes. This description dates back to early medical writings, where ancient Greek physicians, notably Hippocrates, referred to various blinding eye conditions collectively as "glaykoseis" (1). Early Greek texts often lacked specificity, grouping several distinct ocular diseases under broad descriptions, resulting in considerable diagnostic confusion.

During the Roman era, the influential physician Galen continued to perpetuate misconceptions, linking vision impairment primarily with opacities of the crystalline lens rather than recognizing the role of increased intraocular pressure (2). Galen's theories dominated medical thought for centuries, significantly delaying accurate understanding of glaucoma's underlying mechanisms. The historical journey of glaucoma understanding also reveals fascinating regional variations in approaches to treatment. Traditional Chinese medicine, dating back to the Sui Dynasty (581–618), described conditions resembling glaucoma and proposed herbal remedies and acupuncture techniques to address ocular discomfort and vision loss. These practices developed independently from Western medical traditions, emphasizing the balance of energy flow rather than anatomical structures (3).

Throughout the medieval period, limited advancements occurred in glaucoma diagnosis or treatment. The period was characterized by reliance on Galenic principles, with practitioners employing treatments based on humoral balance rather than empirical evidence (2). Notably, the advent of Arabic medicine introduced some ophthalmologic innovations; however, glaucoma was not clearly delineated from other ocular disorders during this era. The Renaissance brought about critical advancements, notably in anatomical understanding and medical dissemination through the printing press. Andreas Vesalius's detailed anatomical dissections paved the way for better ocular understanding, although precise knowledge of glaucoma lagged behind due to persistent confusion with cataracts and other lens-related conditions. Consequently, treatments remained predominantly ineffective and symptomatic, focusing largely on superficial alleviation of discomfort rather than underlying pathophysiology.

A pivotal moment in glaucoma's history occurred in the 17th century with English physician Richard Banister (died in 1626), who noted the characteristic hardening of the eye associated with increased intraocular pressure, marking one of the earliest distinctions of glaucoma as a separate disease entity (Duke-Elder, 1969). Despite Banister's insightful observations, practical therapeutic solutions were slow to emerge. The 18th and early 19th centuries witnessed a gradual evolution in medical approaches to glaucoma, with the recognition of intraocular pressure playing a more central role. The true revolution occurred in 1851, when Hermann von Helmholtz invented the ophthalmoscope, providing clinicians the unprecedented ability to visualize the optic nerve directly. This instrument facilitated the identification of characteristic glaucomatous optic disc cupping, radically enhancing diagnostic capabilities (2, 3). Shortly thereafter, German ophthalmologist Albrecht von Graefe made a monumental advancement by introducing iridectomy in 1856. This surgical procedure, designed to reduce intraocular pressure by creating an opening in the iris, represented the foundation of modern surgical glaucoma treatments (4). These advancements marked the beginning of targeted therapeutic interventions based on physiological insights rather than symptomatic relief alone.

In parallel, pharmacological advancements significantly influenced glaucoma treatment. In 1876, Ludwig Laqueur discovered that physostigmine, derived from the Calabar bean, effectively lowered intraocular pressure, initiating pharmacological management of glaucoma (4). Technological developments continued into the 20th century with the introduction of the Schiotz tonometer, a device that standardized and simplified the measurement of intraocular pressure. The mid-to-late 20th century was marked by further innovations. New classes of glaucoma medications emerged, notably beta-blockers and prostaglandin analogs, significantly improving patient outcomes. Concurrently, surgical interventions evolved substantially with the advent of laser trabeculoplasty and minimally invasive glaucoma surgeries (MIGS), which offered less invasive yet highly effective means of pressure control.

Despite these transformative developments, glaucoma remains a substantial clinical challenge, particularly due to its asymptomatic nature in early stages. Continuous research is thus vital, especially in areas such as genetics, neuroprotection, and improved screening methodologies for early disease detection. Advances in imaging technologies, such as optical coherence tomography (OCT), have also greatly improved diagnostic precision and monitoring capabilities in recent years. Moreover, the social impact of glaucoma throughout history merits consideration. Before effective treatments, glaucoma often resulted in complete blindness, dramatically altering individuals' socioeconomic status and quality of life. Historical records indicate that vision loss due to what we now recognize as glaucoma frequently led to poverty and social marginalization, particularly among working-class populations who relied on visual acuity for employment (5). The 20th century also saw critical paradigm shifts in conceptualizing glaucoma. The disease, initially defined solely by elevated intraocular pressure, underwent significant reclassification when researchers identified patients with normal-tension glaucoma—exhibiting characteristic optic nerve damage despite normal pressure readings. This discovery fundamentally altered the disease definition, moving it from a purely pressure-related condition to a more complex optic neuropathy (6).

The evolution of terminology also reflects our developing understanding. The distinction between primary open-angle glaucoma and angle-closure glaucoma emerged in the early 20th century, with Edward Jackson and other ophthalmologists establishing classification systems that remain foundational to modern practice. This nomenclature evolution paralleled advances in gonioscopy techniques that allowed direct visualization of the anterior chamber angle (7). Another significant but often overlooked milestone was the development of visual field testing methodologies. The introduction of perimetry by Hans Goldmann in the 1940s revolutionized the ability to detect and monitor functional vision loss, providing a quantifiable measure of disease progression that complemented anatomical observations. The narrative of glaucoma research also includes notable failures and detours. Several widely adopted treatments later proved ineffective or harmful, including early approaches such as bloodletting and mercury applications. These historical missteps underscore the importance of evidence-based medicine in contemporary glaucoma management and highlight how scientific progress often advances through trial and error (8).

As we examine glaucoma's historical trajectory, it becomes evident that our current understanding represents the culmination of centuries of observation, innovation, and scientific inquiry—a process that continues today as researchers explore neuroprotective strategies, genetic factors, and biomarkers to further advance glaucoma care in the 21st century. Today, the historical narrative of glaucoma continues to evolve, shaped by ongoing research and clinical advancements. The lessons derived from centuries of observational and empirical experiences underscore the necessity for multidisciplinary approaches and continued innovation to effectively combat glaucoma's global burden.

SECTION 2—EPIDEMIOLOGY: GLOBAL BURDEN AND PUBLIC HEALTH IMPACT

Glaucoma is a major global health concern, affecting millions of individuals and ranking among the leading causes of irreversible blindness. Its silent and progressive nature makes it particularly challenging to detect in its early stages, resulting in late diagnoses and limited treatment options for many patients. Understanding its epidemiology is crucial for public health planning, resource allocation, and early intervention strategies aimed at mitigating its burden on individuals and healthcare systems worldwide. This section explores the prevalence of glaucoma, its demographic and geographic variations, and its broader implications for public health. Glaucoma's prevalence has been increasing, largely due to aging populations and the rise of associated risk factors such as diabetes and hypertension. As of 2013, approximately 64.3 million people worldwide were estimated to have glaucoma, with projections suggesting that this number will rise to 111.8 million by 2040 (9). These estimates highlight the growing impact of glaucoma on global health, particularly in regions with aging populations and limited access to healthcare.

Primary open-angle glaucoma (POAG) is the most common form of the disease, with significant variations in prevalence across different populations. The highest rates of POAG have been observed in Africa, where prevalence reaches approximately 4.20%. In contrast, primary angle-closure glaucoma (PACG) is more predominant in Asia, where prevalence is estimated at 1.09% (9). The disparities in glaucoma types and prevalence highlight the need for region-specific screening programs and treatment strategies. In the United States, more than 3 million Americans are affected by glaucoma, and this number is expected to exceed 6.3 million by 2050 due to the aging population (CDC, 2023). Studies indicate that approximately 50% of glaucoma cases in the U.S. remain undiagnosed, largely due to the asymptomatic nature of the disease in its early stages (Glaucoma Research Foundation, 2023). A study by Ehrlich et al. reported that 4.22 million U.S. adults had glaucoma in 2022, with 1.49 million experiencing significant vision impairment due to the condition (10).

Age remains one of the strongest risk factors for glaucoma, with incidence rates increasing significantly after the age of 40. Gender differences have also been documented; in the United States, an estimated 1.94 million males and 2.29 million females were diagnosed with glaucoma in 2022, indicating a slightly higher prevalence among females (10). However, the gender-based differences vary across different types of glaucoma and ethnic backgrounds.

Ethnic disparities in glaucoma prevalence are well-documented. In the U.S., Black individuals are approximately three times more likely to develop vision-threatening glaucoma compared to White individuals (11). Hispanic populations also face an increased risk, particularly for POAG, which has been linked to genetic and environmental factors. In Asia, where PACG is more common, the condition is often diagnosed at a more advanced stage due to limited awareness and healthcare access.

Geographically, within the U.S., states like Mississippi have the highest glaucoma prevalence, with rates reaching 1.95%, whereas Utah has the lowest prevalence at 1.11%. The variation is attributed to differences in demographics, healthcare access, and the availability of routine eye screenings. The epidemiological landscape of glaucoma is further complicated by the emergence of environmental and lifestyle factors as potential contributors. Urbanization has been associated with higher glaucoma prevalence in several regions, potentially due to increased exposure to air pollution and altered sleep patterns from light pollution. Recent studies indicate that chronic exposure to particulate matter may accelerate optic nerve damage through oxidative stress mechanisms, particularly in genetically susceptible individuals. Additionally, the growing prevalence of myopia worldwide, especially in East Asian populations, presents another concerning trend, as moderate to high myopia significantly increases the risk of developing open-angle glaucoma.

The socioeconomic gradient in glaucoma burden is increasingly evident across various healthcare systems. Even in countries with universal healthcare coverage, lower socioeconomic status correlates with later diagnosis, poorer adherence to treatment regimens, and worse clinical outcomes. This disparity stems from multiple factors, including reduced health literacy, financial barriers to medication access despite insurance coverage, and logistical challenges in maintaining regular ophthalmological appointments. The gradual nature of vision loss in glaucoma often means that socioeconomically disadvantaged patients seek care only when the disease has progressed to advanced stages, significantly limiting treatment efficacy.

Comorbidity patterns also shape the epidemiological profile of glaucoma globally. The increasing prevalence of diabetes mellitus, especially in rapidly developing economies, amplifies glaucoma risk across populations previously showing lower incidence rates. Vascular conditions such as hypertension and cardiovascular disease similarly modify glaucoma risk profiles, creating complex interrelationships that challenge traditional epidemiological categorizations based solely on geographic or ethnic determinants. These evolving patterns necessitate more sophisticated public health approaches that address not only glaucoma in isolation but also its interconnections with the broader spectrum of non-communicable diseases affecting aging populations worldwide.

Globally, limited access to ophthalmologic care remains a major challenge in many developing countries. Africa, despite having the highest prevalence of POAG, has some of the lowest glaucoma detection rates due to insufficient healthcare infrastructure and trained ophthalmologists. In Asia, large-scale screening programs have been implemented in certain countries, but challenges persist in rural regions where access to specialist care remains limited.

Glaucoma imposes a significant economic burden on individuals, healthcare systems, and society as a whole. In the United States, the direct medical costs associated with glaucoma, including diagnostics, medications, and surgical interventions, exceed $2.86 billion annually (12). Indirect costs, such as lost productivity, caregiver burden, and reduced quality of life, further escalate the financial impact of the disease.

The economic impact is even more pronounced in low- and middle-income countries (LMICs), where the cost of glaucoma treatment often exceeds the financial capacity of patients. A lack of affordable medications and surgical interventions leads to a higher prevalence of blindness and disability, further exacerbating poverty and dependence on social support systems (11). Beyond economic costs, glaucoma significantly affects patients' quality of life. Vision loss due to glaucoma limits independence, making daily activities such as driving, reading, and walking challenging. Studies have shown that individuals with glaucoma have higher rates of depression and anxiety due to the progressive nature of the disease and the fear of complete blindness (13). Social withdrawal is common among glaucoma patients, particularly in advanced stages when mobility and functional vision become severely impaired.

Given the silent progression of glaucoma, early detection and intervention are crucial to mitigating its impact. Public health initiatives must focus on the following:

1. *Awareness Campaigns*: Increasing public knowledge about glaucoma, its risk factors, and the importance of regular eye exams. Targeted outreach efforts should focus on high-risk populations, including individuals over 60 and those with a family history of glaucoma.
2. *Screening and Early Diagnosis*: Implementing systematic screening programs, particularly in high-prevalence regions. Community-based screening initiatives using portable tonometry and fundus imaging can improve early detection rates in underserved populations.
3. *Access to Care*: Expanding access to affordable glaucoma treatments, including medications and surgical interventions, especially in LMICs. Governments and health organizations must prioritize funding for eye care services and training programs for ophthalmologists.
4. *Integration with Primary Healthcare*: Strengthening primary healthcare systems to incorporate routine glaucoma screening in standard check-ups. Educating general practitioners on glaucoma symptoms and risk factors can enhance early referrals to specialists.
5. *Telemedicine and AI-Based Diagnostics*: Leveraging telemedicine and artificial intelligence to bridge gaps in eye care accessibility. AI-driven diagnostic tools, such as deep learning algorithms for retinal imaging analysis, have shown promising results in detecting glaucomatous changes at an early stage (10).

To conclude this section, glaucoma presents an escalating public health challenge with profound economic and social implications. Addressing its global burden requires multiple approaches, including early detection, improved access to treatment, and enhanced public awareness. By implementing comprehensive public health strategies and leveraging technological advancements, healthcare systems can work toward reducing glaucoma-related blindness and improving patient outcomes worldwide.

SECTION 3—WHY THIS BOOK? BRIDGING THE GAP BETWEEN SCIENCE AND PRACTICE

The landscape of glaucoma research, diagnostics, and management has witnessed remarkable advancements over the past several decades. From sophisticated imaging technologies to novel pharmacological agents and surgical innovations, the scientific understanding of this complex disease has expanded exponentially. Yet despite these scientific breakthroughs, a concerning disparity persists between the wealth of scientific knowledge and its practical implementation in clinical settings worldwide. This book emerges as a response to this critical gap, aiming to forge meaningful connections between cutting-edge science and everyday clinical practice in glaucoma management.

The divide between scientific knowledge and clinical practice in glaucoma management manifests in several ways. First, there exists a considerable lag time between scientific discovery and clinical implementation. While research publications may report promising new diagnostic approaches or therapeutic interventions, the translation of these findings into standardized clinical protocols often takes years, if not decades. For instance, despite compelling evidence supporting the efficacy of selective laser trabeculoplasty (SLT) as a first-line treatment for open-angle glaucoma, many clinicians continue to initiate treatment with topical medications, adhering to traditional management paradigms rather than evidence-based approaches (14).

Second, the accessibility of scientific knowledge varies dramatically across different healthcare settings. Clinicians in academic medical centers may have ready access to the latest research findings, technological innovations, and multidisciplinary expertise. In contrast, those practicing in community-based settings, particularly in resource-limited environments, often face significant barriers to accessing and implementing current evidence-based practices. The result is a heterogeneous landscape of glaucoma care, where the quality and approach to management may differ substantially depending on geographic location, institutional resources, and individual practitioner awareness.

Third, the complexity of scientific literature itself poses a challenge for busy clinicians. The exponential growth of research publications, often presenting conflicting or nuanced findings, can overwhelm practitioners attempting to distill practical guidelines from the scientific literature. Without clear syntheses of current evidence, clinicians may struggle to determine which innovations warrant adoption into their practice and which require further validation before clinical implementation.

This knowledge-practice gap carries profound implications for patient care. Delayed adoption of evidence-based practices means that many patients do not benefit from optimal management strategies in a timely manner. The variability in care approaches contributes to health disparities, with certain populations receiving outdated or suboptimal treatments based solely on where they receive care. Furthermore, the underutilization of proven diagnostic and therapeutic advances represents a missed opportunity to mitigate the personal and societal burden of vision loss from glaucoma.

From a public health perspective, the knowledge-practice gap also impacts resource allocation and healthcare economics. Inefficient diagnostic approaches and treatment strategies that fail to halt disease progression ultimately lead to increased healthcare utilization, as patients with advanced glaucoma require more intensive interventions and support services. The economic burden extends beyond direct healthcare costs to include productivity losses, caregiver burden, and reduced quality of life—consequences that might be mitigated through more effective translation of scientific knowledge into clinical practice.

This book aims to address the knowledge-practice divide through a multi-dimensional approach designed to make scientific advances accessible, applicable, and actionable for clinicians across diverse practice settings. Rather than simply presenting scientific findings in isolation, it contextualizes research within clinical scenarios, providing clear pathways for implementation even in resource-constrained environments.

A fundamental premise of this work is that understanding the basic science underlying glaucoma is essential for optimal clinical decision-making. Each chapter therefore begins with core scientific concepts—whether anatomical, physiological, or pathological—and systematically builds toward their clinical applications. For example, discussions of aqueous humor dynamics move beyond theoretical descriptions to explore how these mechanisms inform therapeutic targets and explain medication efficacies. Similarly, examinations of optic nerve structure and function connect directly to diagnostic approaches and monitoring strategies. This integrative approach serves multiple purposes. For researchers and academic clinicians, it reinforces the clinical relevance of scientific investigations. For community-based practitioners, it provides the scientific rationale that underpins clinical protocols, enabling more informed adaptation to individual patient scenarios. For trainees, it establishes a foundation of understanding that bridges the often-siloed worlds of basic science and clinical medicine.

Recognizing the global nature of glaucoma and the vast differences in healthcare resources worldwide, this book deliberately addresses implementation across diverse practice settings. Where sophisticated diagnostic technologies are discussed, the text also explores alternative approaches for resource-limited environments. When describing surgical techniques, considerations for settings with limited access to specialized equipment or postoperative care are included. Pharmacological discussions acknowledge issues of medication cost, availability, and compliance that may vary across geographic and socioeconomic contexts. This pragmatic approach reflects an understanding that the goal of bridging science and practice must account for real-world constraints. Rather than presenting an idealized version of glaucoma management accessible only to well-resourced institutions, the book offers tiered approaches that allow clinicians to provide the best possible care within their particular constraints while working toward optimal standards.

The overwhelming volume of scientific literature presents a significant barrier for clinicians seeking to incorporate current evidence into their practice. This book addresses this challenge by providing carefully synthesized summaries of evidence across key domains of glaucoma management. Rather than simply cataloging research findings, it critically evaluates the quality of evidence, highlighting areas of consensus, controversy, and ongoing investigation. This critical evaluation extends to new and emerging technologies. While acknowledging the excitement surrounding innovations such as artificial intelligence-assisted diagnostics, sustained-release drug delivery systems, and novel surgical devices, the book maintains a balanced perspective on their current limitations and evidence gaps. This approach helps clinicians distinguish between technologies ready for clinical adoption and those requiring further validation, protecting patients from the risks of prematurely implemented interventions while ensuring they benefit from genuinely advantageous advances.

The knowledge-practice gap in glaucoma management affects a wide range of stakeholders beyond just clinicians and researchers. This book acknowledges this broader impact by including perspectives relevant to patients, healthcare administrators, policymakers, and educators. Understanding that effective glaucoma management ultimately depends on patient engagement and adherence, the book incorporates patient perspectives throughout. Chapter 11, focuses entirely on living with glaucoma, amplifies patient voices through personal narratives that illuminate the lived experience of the disease. These accounts serve not only to humanize the scientific and clinical discussions but also to highlight practical challenges in treatment adherence, adaptation to visual impairment, and psychological coping that may not be apparent from a purely medical perspective. Additionally, discussions of diagnostic and therapeutic approaches include considerations of patient experience, preferences, and quality of life impacts. This patient-centered orientation reminds practitioners that bridging science and practice ultimately means translating scientific advances into meaningful benefits for individuals living with glaucoma or at risk of developing the disease.

Effective translation of scientific knowledge into clinical practice often requires systemic changes beyond individual practitioner behavior. Acknowledging this reality, the book addresses organizational, economic, and policy factors that influence glaucoma care delivery. Chapter 9, focuses on public health aspects of glaucoma, examines screening program implementation, healthcare access barriers, and resource allocation decisions that shape population-level outcomes. These discussions provide valuable context for healthcare administrators and policymakers seeking to optimize glaucoma care systems. By explaining the scientific rationale underlying recommendations for systemic changes, the book helps bridge another critical gap: that between clinical evidence and healthcare policy. Recent research generally highlights the importance of such approaches, demonstrating that multidimensional interventions that address both provider and system-level factors are most effective in improving glaucoma care delivery and patient outcomes.

Recognizing that sustainable improvements in glaucoma management require changes in how future practitioners are trained, the book incorporates educational perspectives throughout. Case studies are structured not merely to illustrate clinical scenarios but to model clinical reasoning processes that integrate scientific knowledge with patient-specific factors. Diagnostic and management algorithms are presented as decision-making frameworks rather than rigid protocols, encouraging adaptive thinking that can respond to both scientific advances and individual patient circumstances. This educational orientation makes the book valuable not only as a reference for established practitioners but also as a teaching tool for ophthalmology residency programs, optometry schools, and continuing education contexts. By modeling how to integrate science and practice from the earliest stages of professional development, the book contributes to long-term narrowing of the knowledge-practice gap.

While we make comprehensive effort to bridge the gap between science and practice in glaucoma management, we acknowledge that this bridge must be dynamic rather than static. The field continues to evolve rapidly, with ongoing research constantly refining our understanding of disease mechanisms, risk factors, diagnostic approaches, and treatment efficacies. New technologies emerge, existing therapies are reevaluated, and patient populations change in their demographics and expectations.

In this context, the book serves not as a definitive endpoint but as a foundation for continued engagement with evolving evidence. Its frameworks for critical evaluation of new findings, its emphasis on fundamental principles that transcend specific technologies or techniques, and its attention to implementation science provide readers with tools to maintain the science-practice bridge even as the landscape on both sides continues to shift. The ultimate measure of this book's success will be its contribution to improved patient outcomes through more effective, equitable, and evidence-based glaucoma care. By providing a comprehensive yet accessible integration of scientific knowledge and clinical application, it aims to empower clinicians, researchers, patients, administrators, and policymakers to work collectively toward reducing the burden of glaucoma-related vision loss worldwide. In bridging the gap between what is known and what is practiced, it seeks to fulfill the fundamental promise of medical science: the translation of understanding into healing.

CHAPTER 2
ANATOMY AND
PHYSIOLOGY OF
THE EYE

The human eye is one of the most complex and finely tuned organs in the body, allowing us to perceive and interpret the world around us. Its complex structure and physiological processes work harmoniously to enable vision, making any disturbance in its function a matter of significant concern. In the context of glaucoma, understanding the anatomy and physiology of the eye is crucial for comprehending how this disease develops, progresses, and ultimately leads to vision loss. This chapter provides a foundational overview of the eye's structure, the dynamics of aqueous humor and intraocular pressure (IOP), and the optic nerve's vital role in visual processing.

The first section, "The Eye's Structure: A Foundation for Understanding Glaucoma," delves into the anatomy of the eye, highlighting key components that are relevant to the pathophysiology of glaucoma. The eye's various structures—including the cornea, lens, ciliary body, trabecular meshwork, and retina—each play distinct roles in vision and ocular health. Particular emphasis will be placed on the anterior chamber, where aqueous humor is produced and drained, as any disruption in this balance is a primary contributor to glaucoma. The interaction between these structures is essential in maintaining clear vision and ensuring proper ocular function.

In the second section, "Aqueous Humor Dynamics and Intraocular Pressure (IOP)," the focus shifts to the fluid dynamics within the eye. Aqueous humor, the clear fluid that nourishes the eye and maintains intraocular pressure, is central to glaucoma development. The balance between aqueous humor production by the ciliary body and its drainage through the trabecular meshwork and uveoscleral outflow pathways determines IOP. Increased resistance to outflow or excessive production can elevate intraocular pressure, leading to progressive optic nerve damage. This section will discuss the physiological mechanisms governing aqueous humor circulation, regulatory factors influencing IOP, and how these processes become dysregulated in glaucoma.

The third section, "The Optic Nerve and Visual Pathway," examines the role of the optic nerve in transmitting visual information from the eye to the brain. The optic nerve is particularly vulnerable to damage in glaucoma, as elevated intraocular pressure and other pathological mechanisms contribute to retinal ganglion cell loss and axonal degeneration. This section explores the structure and function of the optic nerve, the visual pathway from the retina to the visual cortex, and the impact of glaucoma-related damage on visual fields. Additionally, the discussion will address the mechanisms of neurodegeneration, potential protective strategies, and emerging research aimed at preserving optic nerve health.

By understanding the anatomy and physiology of the eye, we gain essential insights into the mechanisms underlying glaucoma. This knowledge not only informs

DOI: 10.1201/9781003646693-2

diagnosis and treatment strategies but also highlights areas for further research and innovation in preventing and managing this sight-threatening disease. The following sections will provide a deeper exploration of these fundamental concepts, offering a comprehensive perspective on the eye's structure, its physiological processes, and their relationship to glaucoma pathology.

SECTION I—THE EYE'S STRUCTURE— A FOUNDATION FOR UNDERSTANDING GLAUCOMA

The human eye is a highly specialized organ that captures and processes visual information, allowing us to perceive the world around us. Its complex anatomical structures and physiological processes work in concert to maintain clear vision, and any disruption in this delicate system can lead to significant visual impairment. Glaucoma, one of the leading causes of blindness worldwide, primarily affects the optic nerve, but its pathogenesis is deeply intertwined with the structural and functional integrity of multiple ocular components. Understanding the anatomy of the eye is therefore essential for grasping how glaucoma develops, progresses, and leads to irreversible vision loss. This section provides a comprehensive overview of the anatomical structures of the eye, with a focus on those most relevant to glaucoma.

Figure 2.1 presents a clear visualization of the eye's anatomy. The outermost structures of the eye serve protective functions and contribute to the overall

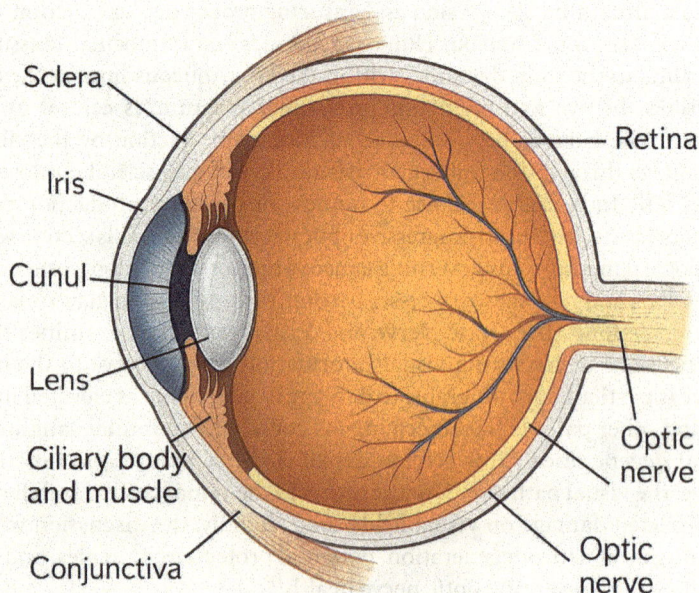

Figure 2.1 Sketch of the eye's anatomy.

integrity of the visual system. The sclera, or the white, opaque outer layer, maintains the shape of the eye and acts as a protective barrier against mechanical injury and microbial invasion. Its fibrous nature ensures that the internal structures remain stable, despite constant exposure to environmental elements (15). At the front of the eye, the cornea serves as a transparent, dome-shaped window that refracts light onto the retina. Unlike the sclera, the cornea lacks blood vessels, relying instead on the aqueous humor and tear film for nourishment. The conjunctiva, a thin mucous membrane covering the sclera and the inside of the eyelids, provides additional protection by lubricating the eye and preventing infections.

The anterior segment of the eye consists of the anterior and posterior chambers, which are filled with aqueous humor—a clear fluid crucial for maintaining intraocular pressure and nourishing avascular structures such as the cornea and lens. The iris, the pigmented structure responsible for regulating the amount of light entering the eye, separates these two chambers.

Aqueous humor is produced by the ciliary body, a specialized tissue located behind the iris, and circulates through the pupil before draining via the trabecular meshwork and Schlemm's canal. Any disruption in this drainage system can lead to increased resistance to outflow, resulting in elevated IOP—a key risk factor for glaucoma. Primary open-angle glaucoma (POAG) is characterized by dysfunction in the trabecular meshwork, leading to gradual IOP elevation and subsequent optic nerve damage (16). On the other hand, primary angle-closure glaucoma (PACG) occurs when the peripheral iris obstructs the trabecular meshwork, preventing aqueous humor from escaping the anterior chamber and causing acute spikes in IOP (17).

Positioned directly behind the iris, the lens is a transparent, biconvex structure that focuses light onto the retina. The lens is held in place by suspensory ligaments, which attach to the ciliary body. Over time, changes in the lens's position and shape may contribute to narrow-angle glaucoma, particularly in older adults, as the lens thickens and pushes the iris forward, exacerbating angle closure (18). This highlights the interdependence of ocular structures and their collective role in maintaining proper fluid dynamics within the eye.

The posterior segment of the eye includes the vitreous chamber, retina, choroid, and optic nerve, all of which are critical for visual function. The retina is a highly specialized neural tissue that converts light into electrical signals. It contains two types of photoreceptors: rods, which enable vision in low light, and cones, which facilitate color vision and high-resolution central vision. At the center of the retina lies the macula, responsible for fine detail and sharp central vision. Within the macula, the fovea contains the highest concentration of cone cells, making it the most sensitive part of the retina.

Beneath the retina, the choroid serves as a vascular layer that supplies oxygen and nutrients to retinal cells. Reduced blood flow to the choroid has been implicated in glaucomatous damage, as ischemia and oxidative stress contribute to retinal ganglion cell apoptosis (19). The optic nerve, often considered the primary site of glaucomatous damage, carries visual information from the retina to the brain. It is composed of over a million retinal ganglion cell axons, which converge at the optic nerve head (optic disc). This region is particularly vulnerable to the effects of elevated IOP, as mechanical compression and ischemic stress can lead to progressive axonal degeneration. Clinically, this manifests as optic nerve cupping, a hallmark of glaucoma that results from the loss of neural tissue and excavation of the optic disc (15).

Emerging research suggests that glaucomatous damage is not solely due to elevated IOP but also involves vascular dysregulation and impaired ocular blood flow. The ophthalmic artery supplies blood to the eye, with branches reaching the retina, optic nerve, and choroid. Dysregulation of these vascular networks, often observed in normal-tension glaucoma (NTG), may lead to insufficient perfusion of the optic nerve, contributing to progressive nerve fiber loss despite normal IOP levels (20). Studies indicate that systemic conditions such as hypertension and diabetes can exacerbate vascular compromise, increasing the risk of glaucomatous progression in susceptible individuals (18).

The lamina cribrosa, a specialized connective tissue structure at the optic nerve head, deserves particular attention in the context of glaucoma. This mesh-like structure provides support for retinal ganglion cell axons as they exit the eye, creating a potential anatomical vulnerability. Research has shown that the lamina cribrosa undergoes significant remodeling in glaucomatous eyes, including posterior displacement, compression, and altered biomechanical properties (21). These changes may exacerbate axonal damage by creating mechanical stress and impeding axoplasmic flow, essential for transporting nutrients and cellular components to maintain neural health. Individual variations in lamina cribrosa architecture and biomechanical properties may explain the differential susceptibility to glaucomatous damage among patients with similar IOP levels (22). Advanced imaging techniques, including enhanced-depth imaging optical coherence tomography (EDI-OCT), have enabled in vivo visualization of the lamina cribrosa, offering new insights into its role in glaucoma pathogenesis and potentially serving as a biomarker for disease progression and treatment response.

The complex anatomy of the eye directly influences treatment strategies for glaucoma. Traditional medical approaches target the physiological processes of aqueous humor dynamics—topical medications may decrease aqueous humor production (beta-blockers, carbonic anhydrase inhibitors), increase conventional outflow (miotics, Rho-kinase inhibitors), or enhance uveoscleral outflow (prostaglandin analogs). Surgical interventions similarly exploit anatomical pathways: trabeculectomy creates an alternative drainage route for aqueous humor, while minimally invasive glaucoma surgeries (MIGS) aim to enhance outflow through Schlemm's canal or establish new drainage pathways with less tissue disruption. Novel approaches target neuroprotection of retinal ganglion cells and their axons, acknowledging that glaucoma damage extends beyond pressure-related mechanisms. Anatomical variations among patients, including differences in anterior chamber depth, angle configuration, and trabecular meshwork architecture, necessitate personalized treatment approaches. Furthermore, age-related changes in ocular structures—such as lens thickening, decreased trabecular meshwork cellularity, and altered extracellular matrix composition—may impact both disease progression and treatment efficacy. Understanding these anatomical nuances allows clinicians to tailor interventions to individual patients, potentially improving outcomes and slowing disease progression.

Table 2.1 Key Anatomical Structures of the Eye Relevant to Glaucoma

Structure	Location	Function Relevant to Glaucoma	Clinical Relevance in Glaucoma
Trabecular Meshwork	Anterior chamber angle	Drains aqueous humor into Schlemm's canal	Main site of outflow resistance in POAG
Schlemm's Canal	Adjacent to trabecular meshwork	Collects aqueous humor from trabecular meshwork	Targeted in MIGS procedures
Ciliary Body	Posterior to iris	Produces aqueous humor	Target of beta-blockers & carbonic anhydrase inhibitors
Optic Nerve Head	Posterior pole of eye	Transmits visual signals to brain	Main site of glaucomatous damage
Lamina Cribrosa	Within optic nerve head	Supports optic nerve fibers	Vulnerable to IOP-induced stress
Iris	Anterior chamber	Regulates pupil size; impacts angle width	Iris crowding in PACG
Anterior Chamber Angle	Between cornea & iris	Determines accessibility of outflow pathway	Determines glaucoma subtype (open vs. closed)

This section aimed to justify that a clear understanding of ocular anatomy is crucial for appreciating how glaucoma develops and progresses. Table 2.1 summarizes the key anatomical structures of the eye that play a central role in the pathogenesis, diagnosis, and treatment of glaucoma, highlighting their locations, primary functions, and clinical significance.

To conclude this section, the eye's anatomy plays a crucial role in the development and progression of glaucoma. From the aqueous humor dynamics in the anterior segment to the structural vulnerability of the optic nerve, multiple interconnected components contribute to the disease's pathophysiology. Understanding these anatomical and physiological aspects is essential for diagnosing glaucoma, developing effective treatments, and implementing preventive strategies. As research advances, new insights into ocular blood flow, neuroprotection, and innovative surgical interventions will continue to shape the future of glaucoma.

SECTION 2—AQUEOUS HUMOR DYNAMICS AND INTRAOCULAR PRESSURE (IOP)

Intraocular pressure (IOP) represents one of the most critical physiological parameters in ophthalmology and serves as the primary modifiable risk factor in glaucoma management. The delicate balance that maintains IOP within normal limits depends on the continuous production, circulation, and drainage of aqueous humor—a clear fluid that fills the anterior and posterior chambers of the eye. This section explores the mechanisms governing aqueous humor dynamics, the factors influencing IOP regulation, and how disruptions in these processes contribute to glaucomatous pathology.

Aqueous humor is actively produced by the ciliary body, a specialized structure located behind the iris in the posterior chamber. The ciliary processes, which consist of approximately 70–80 finger-like projections, contain a rich network of fenestrated capillaries surrounded by a double-layered epithelium (23). The non-pigmented ciliary epithelium, which faces the posterior chamber, is primarily responsible for aqueous humor secretion through a combination of active transport mechanisms, ultrafiltration, and passive diffusion. The process of aqueous humor formation begins with plasma ultrafiltration from the capillaries of the ciliary processes. However, the composition of aqueous humor differs significantly from that of plasma, indicating that active secretory processes play a predominant role. The non-pigmented ciliary epithelium contains numerous mitochondria and membrane-bound enzymes, particularly Na^+/K^+-ATPase, which facilitate the selective transport of ions across the blood–aqueous barrier. This active transport creates osmotic gradients that drive water movement into the posterior chamber.

Several key biochemical pathways contribute to aqueous humor production. Carbonic anhydrase catalyzes the formation of bicarbonate ions, which are actively transported into the posterior chamber alongside sodium ions. This process creates an electrochemical gradient that promotes the passive flow of water, chloride, and other solutes. Additionally, specific transport proteins mediate the movement of ascorbate, amino acids, and other essential nutrients into the aqueous humor, while preventing the entry of larger molecules like proteins under normal conditions.

The rate of aqueous humor production averages approximately 2.5–2.8 µL/minute in healthy adults, resulting in a turnover rate of about 1% of the anterior chamber volume per minute (24). This production follows a circadian rhythm, with higher rates during waking hours and decreased production during sleep—a pattern that explains the typical diurnal variation in IOP measurements. Numerous factors can influence this production rate, including age, systemic blood pressure, hormonal status, and pharmacological interventions. Once secreted into the posterior chamber, aqueous humor flows around the lens and through the pupil into the anterior chamber. This circulatory pattern is driven by convection currents generated by temperature differences between the relatively warm iris and the cooler cornea, as well as by the continuous production-drainage dynamics.

Aqueous humor serves several vital functions beyond establishing IOP. First, it provides nutritional support to avascular structures, including the corneal endothelium, trabecular meshwork, and lens. It supplies glucose, amino acids, and oxygen while removing metabolic waste products. Second, it contributes to the optical clarity of the eye by maintaining precise hydration levels in the cornea. Third, it creates a physiologically stable environment by regulating pH and electrolyte balance. Fourth, it contains specific growth factors and cytokines that may influence the health and function of anterior segment tissues. Finally, it participates in immunological processes through the presence of complement components and immunoglobulins, albeit at significantly lower concentrations than in serum. The composition of aqueous humor reflects its multiple roles. It contains high levels of ascorbate (vitamin C), which may provide antioxidant protection, and specific proteins like transferrin for metal ion transport. The aqueous humor of glaucomatous eyes often shows altered biochemical profiles, including changes in oxidative stress markers, neurotrophic factors, and inflammatory mediators, suggesting that compositional changes may contribute to or result from pathological processes.

The maintenance of normal IOP depends on a balance between aqueous humor production and drainage. Two primary outflow pathways facilitate aqueous humor exit from the anterior chamber: the conventional (trabecular) pathway and the unconventional (uveoscleral) pathway.

The conventional pathway accounts for approximately 80–90% of aqueous humor drainage in healthy eyes. This route involves sequential passage through the trabecular meshwork, Schlemm's canal, collector channels, and episcleral veins before ultimately reaching the venous circulation (25). The trabecular meshwork consists of three distinct regions: the uveal meshwork, the corneoscleral meshwork, and the juxtacanalicular tissue (JCT). The JCT, which lies adjacent to Schlemm's canal, provides the greatest resistance to aqueous outflow and is therefore the primary site determining outflow facility.

The trabecular meshwork is not merely a passive filter but a metabolically active tissue that can modulate its resistance characteristics. Trabecular meshwork cells synthesize and degrade extracellular matrix components, phagocytose debris, and respond to mechanical and biochemical signals to regulate outflow resistance. These cells express contractile proteins and receptors for various mediators, allowing dynamic adjustments to outflow facility. For instance, trabecular meshwork cells can contract in response to endothelin-1 and relax in response to nitric oxide, thereby modulating the spaces between trabecular beams. The endothelial cells lining Schlemm's canal also play an active role in aqueous humor drainage. These cells form giant vacuoles and transcellular pores in response to pressure gradients, facilitating the passage of aqueous humor from the trabecular meshwork into the canal lumen. Once in Schlemm's canal, aqueous humor flows through collector channels and aqueous veins to reach episcleral veins, where it mixes with blood at pressures of approximately 8–10 mmHg (25). The unconventional or uveoscleral pathway provides an alternative route for aqueous humor drainage. This pathway involves fluid movement across the ciliary muscle, through the supraciliary and suprachoroidal spaces, and ultimately into the lymphatic vessels and veins of the orbital tissues. Unlike the conventional pathway, the uveoscleral route does not involve a specialized drainage structure and is less pressure-dependent. In humans, this pathway typically accounts for 10–20% of total outflow, though this proportion can vary with age and in response to certain medications, particularly prostaglandin analogs (26).

Intraocular pressure represents the balance between aqueous humor production and drainage. In healthy adults, IOP typically ranges from 10–21 mmHg, with a mean value of approximately 15–16 mmHg. However, this seemingly narrow range can vary significantly based on numerous factors. IOP demonstrates characteristic diurnal fluctuations, with peak pressures often occurring in the early morning and lowest values recorded during sleep. This pattern primarily reflects changes in aqueous humor production rates, though postural effects and variations in episcleral venous pressure also contribute. The magnitude of these fluctuations can be clinically significant, particularly in glaucoma patients, where larger IOP fluctuations correlate with disease progression. Several physiological mechanisms contribute to IOP regulation. Neural control via sympathetic and parasympathetic innervation influences both aqueous production and drainage. Sympathetic stimulation activates beta-adrenergic receptors in the ciliary epithelium, increasing aqueous production, while alpha-adrenergic stimulation can decrease outflow resistance. Parasympathetic activation contracts the ciliary muscle, which can enhance uveoscleral outflow and also affect conventional outflow by altering trabecular meshwork configuration. Hormonal factors also influence IOP. Corticosteroids are known to increase IOP in susceptible individuals by inducing changes in the trabecular meshwork, including increased deposition of extracellular matrix and reduced phagocytic activity. Thyroid hormones, sex hormones, and growth factors can similarly affect aqueous dynamics, explaining some of the IOP variations observed during pregnancy, menstrual cycles, and endocrine disorders.

Local autoregulatory mechanisms within the eye help maintain IOP homeostasis despite fluctuations in systemic parameters. These mechanisms involve the production of vasoactive substances, cytokines, and metalloproteinases that modulate trabecular meshwork resistance. For example, mechanical stretching of trabecular meshwork cells induces the expression of matrix metalloproteinases (MMPs), which degrade extracellular matrix components, potentially reducing outflow resistance in response to elevated IOP. Disruptions in aqueous humor dynamics represent the primary mechanism underlying IOP elevation in glaucoma. In primary open-angle glaucoma (POAG), the most common form, increased resistance within the conventional outflow pathway leads to progressive IOP elevation despite normal anterior chamber anatomy. Histopathological studies of trabecular meshwork from POAG patients reveal characteristic changes, including decreased cellularity, increased extracellular matrix deposition, particularly in the JCT region, and structural alterations in Schlemm's canal. Multiple mechanisms contribute to this increased outflow resistance. Age-related changes in the trabecular meshwork, including decreased cellularity and altered extracellular matrix composition, may represent a baseline risk factor. Oxidative stress damages trabecular meshwork cells and their cellular components, impairing normal function. Abnormal protein accumulation, including glycosaminoglycans, fibronectin, and other extracellular matrix proteins, narrows the outflow channels. Additionally, impaired trabecular meshwork cell phagocytosis leads to accumulation of debris within the outflow pathways.

In primary angle-closure glaucoma (PACG), anatomical factors physically obstruct aqueous humor access to the trabecular meshwork. These factors include a shallow anterior chamber, narrow iridocorneal angle, and specific iris configurations. In acute angle-closure, pupillary block creates a pressure differential between the posterior and anterior chambers, pushing the peripheral iris forward to occlude the trabecular meshwork. In chronic angle-closure, progressive peripheral anterior synechiae form between the iris and trabecular meshwork, permanently restricting outflow.

Secondary glaucomas involve diverse mechanisms affecting aqueous dynamics. Exfoliative material, pigment particles, inflammatory cells, or neovascular membranes can obstruct the trabecular meshwork. Steroid-induced glaucoma results from

Table 2.2 Aqueous Humor Dynamics: Production vs. Outflow Pathways

Process	Site	Mechanism	Clinical Notes
Production	Ciliary body	Active secretion (Na^+/K^+ ATPase, carbonic anhydrase)	Inhibited by anti-glaucoma medications
Conventional Outflow	Trabecular meshwork → Schlemm's canal	Pressure-dependent	Impaired in POAG
Uveoscleral Outflow	Ciliary muscle → Sclera	Pressure-independent	Enhanced by prostaglandin analogs

trabecular meshwork changes similar to those seen in POAG but accelerated by corticosteroid exposure. Post-traumatic glaucoma may involve angle recession, which damages collector channels and reduces outflow facility.

Normal-tension glaucoma presents a unique challenge to the pressure-centric view of glaucoma pathophysiology. In these patients, optic nerve damage occurs despite IOP measurements within the statistically normal range. This suggests that factors beyond absolute IOP levels, such as IOP fluctuations, vascular dysregulation, or enhanced susceptibility of the optic nerve to pressure effects, contribute significantly to glaucomatous damage.

Since IOP regulation is fundamentally dependent on the dynamic balance between aqueous humor production and outflow, Table 2.2 provides a structured overview of these physiological processes. It distinguishes between the conventional (trabecular) and unconventional (uveoscleral) outflow pathways, while emphasizing their mechanisms and clinical implications in glaucoma management.

Concluding this section, aqueous humor dynamics represent a complex physiological system critical for maintaining ocular health and function. The balance between production and drainage determines IOP, which remains the primary modifiable risk factor in glaucoma management. Understanding these processes provides the foundation for current therapeutic approaches, most of which aim to reduce IOP by either decreasing aqueous humor production or enhancing its outflow. As research advances, new insights into the molecular mechanisms governing trabecular meshwork function, the role of extracellular matrix turnover, and the influence of cytokines and growth factors will likely lead to novel therapeutic targets. Additionally, enhanced understanding of IOP fluctuations, the role of vascular factors, and individual variations in susceptibility to pressure-induced damage will facilitate more personalized approaches to glaucoma management. Through continued investigation of aqueous humor dynamics, we move closer to comprehensive strategies for preserving vision in patients with this sight-threatening disease.

SECTION 3—THE OPTIC NERVE AND VISUAL PATHWAY

The optic nerve represents the critical conduit for visual information transmission from the retina to the brain. In glaucoma, progressive damage to this structure constitutes the fundamental pathology that leads to irreversible vision loss.

Understanding the anatomy, physiology, and vulnerability of the optic nerve and visual pathway provides essential insights into glaucoma's nature, progression, and management. This section examines the optic nerve structure, its connections within the central nervous system, the mechanisms of neurodegeneration in glaucoma, and emerging concepts in neuroprotection. The optic nerve, classified as the second cranial nerve, extends approximately 50 mm from the posterior globe to the optic chiasm. Its unique composition and organization reflect its developmental origin as an extension of the central nervous system rather than a peripheral nerve. The nerve consists of approximately 1.2 million retinal ganglion cell (RGC) axons, which are organized in a topographic fashion that preserves the spatial relationships established in the retina (27).

Anatomically, the optic nerve is divided into four distinct segments: intraocular, intraorbital, intracanalicular, and intracranial. The intraocular portion, commonly referred to as the optic nerve head or optic disc, represents the collection point where RGC axons converge before exiting the eye. This region is clinically visible during ophthalmoscopic examination and displays characteristic changes in glaucoma. The optic nerve head exhibits a complex three-dimensional architecture, comprising several layers from anterior to posterior: the surface nerve fiber layer, the prelaminar region, the laminar region, and the retrolaminar region. The surface nerve fiber layer contains unmyelinated axons that converge from the retina. The prelaminar region, situated between the surface layer and the lamina cribrosa, contains axons arranged in bundles separated by astrocytes and capillaries. The lamina cribrosa, a mesh-like collagenous structure, provides structural support for axon bundles as they exit the eye through openings called laminar pores. This region represents a mechanical and vascular watershed zone, making it particularly vulnerable to pressure-related damage. In the retrolaminar region, axons acquire myelin sheaths from oligodendrocytes, increasing the nerve diameter and changing its physiological properties. The intraorbital segment of the optic nerve follows an S-shaped course within the orbit, allowing for eye movements without tension. This portion is surrounded by cerebrospinal fluid within the subarachnoid space and receives blood supply primarily from branches of the ophthalmic artery. The intracanalicular segment passes through the optic canal in the sphenoid bone, a region where compression can occur in certain pathological conditions. Finally, the intracranial segment extends from the optic canal to the chiasm, lying above the cavernous sinus and internal carotid artery.

From the optic nerve, visual information proceeds posteriorly through a sophisticated neural network. At the optic chiasm, axons from the nasal retina (temporal visual field) cross to the contralateral side, while those from the temporal retina (nasal visual field) continue ipsilaterally. This partial decussation ensures that visual information from each hemifield is processed in the contralateral cerebral hemisphere. Post-chiasmal fibers form the optic tracts, which terminate primarily in the lateral geniculate nucleus (LGN) of the thalamus. The LGN maintains the retinotopic organization of visual information across its six distinct layers. From the LGN, third-order neurons form the optic radiations, with superior fibers projecting directly to the visual cortex and inferior fibers taking a longer course through the temporal lobe (Meyer's loop) before reaching their cortical destinations.

The primary visual cortex (V1), located in the occipital lobe, receives these projections and initiates higher-order visual processing. From V1, information proceeds to specialized visual association areas responsible for analyzing motion, color, form, and other visual attributes. This hierarchical processing creates the complex visual perception we experience (28).

In glaucoma, understanding the visual pathway organization allows clinicians to interpret characteristic visual field defects. For instance, early glaucomatous damage typically affects specific axon bundles in the superior and inferior poles of the optic nerve, resulting in arcuate scotomas that respect the horizontal meridian. Advanced disease may produce "tunnel vision" as peripheral fibers are progressively damaged, while end-stage disease can eliminate all light perception when macular fibers are eventually affected.

Glaucomatous optic neuropathy involves the selective loss of RGCs and their axons, leading to characteristic structural changes at the optic nerve head and corresponding functional visual field loss. Multiple pathophysiological mechanisms contribute to this degenerative process, with elevated IOP historically considered the primary instigating factor. Mechanical forces at the optic nerve head play a significant role in glaucomatous damage. Elevated IOP creates a pressure gradient across the lamina cribrosa, resulting in posterior displacement, compression, and shearing forces that affect axonal transport. These disruptions impede the bidirectional movement of essential cellular components, including mitochondria, neurotrophic factors, and cytoskeletal elements, leading to axonal compromise and eventual degeneration. Vascular factors complement these mechanical mechanisms. Reduced blood flow to the optic nerve head, resulting from either elevated IOP compressing the microvasculature or primary vascular dysregulation, leads to ischemia and reperfusion injury. This process generates reactive oxygen species that damage cellular components and trigger apoptotic cascades. The concept of vascular-related damage helps explain the occurrence of normal-tension glaucoma and the influence of systemic vascular diseases on glaucoma progression.

At the cellular level, glaucomatous damage triggers a cascade of events leading to RGC apoptosis. Mitochondrial dysfunction, oxidative stress, excitotoxicity, and neuroinflammation represent interconnected processes that contribute to neuronal death. Deficient neurotrophic support, particularly brain-derived neurotrophic factor (BDNF), may further compromise RGC survival. Recent evidence suggests that these processes can propagate through trans-neuronal degeneration, affecting structures beyond the primary site of injury, including the LGN and visual cortex.

The selective vulnerability of specific RGC populations represents another intriguing aspect of glaucomatous pathophysiology. Studies indicate that large-diameter RGCs with magnocellular projections, responsible for motion detection and contrast sensitivity, may be preferentially affected early in the disease. This selective vulnerability explains certain patterns of visual dysfunction that precede detectable visual field losses in standard perimetry.

While IOP reduction remains the mainstay of glaucoma treatment, the recognition that neurodegeneration can continue despite IOP control has spurred interest in neuroprotective strategies. These approaches aim to preserve RGC function and survival independent of IOP modulation.

Several neuroprotective targets have emerged from basic science research. Neurotrophic factors, particularly BDNF, have demonstrated protective effects on RGCs in experimental models. Antioxidants that neutralize reactive oxygen species, anti-excitotoxic agents that block excessive glutamate activity, and anti-apoptotic compounds that interfere with programmed cell death pathways represent promising therapeutic avenues. Additionally, approaches targeting neuroinflammation, mitochondrial dysfunction, and protein misfolding have shown potential in preclinical studies.

The concept of neuroregeneration—stimulating damaged RGCs to regrow their axons and reestablish functional connections—represents the frontier of glaucoma research. While the mammalian central nervous system demonstrates limited regenerative capacity, manipulating intrinsic growth programs, modifying inhibitory environmental factors, and utilizing stem cell-based approaches offer hope for future restorative therapies. The optic nerve and visual pathway constitute the neural substrate affected by glaucoma. Understanding their anatomy, physiology, and vulnerability provides critical insights into the nature of glaucomatous damage and informs approaches to diagnosis, monitoring, and treatment. As research advances our understanding of the complex mechanisms underlying RGC death, new therapeutic paradigms will emerge, potentially transforming glaucoma from a progressive, irreversible condition to one where vision preservation and restoration become achievable goals.

CHAPTER 3
PATHOPHYSIOLOGY
OF GLAUCOMA

Glaucoma is a complex and multifactorial disease that leads to progressive damage of the optic nerve and, if left untreated, irreversible vision loss. The pathophysiology of glaucoma involves several mechanisms that include elevated intraocular pressure (IOP), vascular dysregulation, oxidative stress, neuroinflammation, and genetic predisposition. While IOP remains the most significant modifiable risk factor, the disease process extends far beyond simple mechanical pressure, involving a cascade of cellular and molecular events that contribute to retinal ganglion cell apoptosis. Understanding these underlying mechanisms is essential for developing targeted therapeutic strategies and improving patient outcomes.

The first section, "Mechanisms of Optic Nerve Damage," explores the various biological processes that contribute to glaucomatous optic neuropathy. While elevated IOP has historically been considered the primary driver of optic nerve damage, emerging evidence highlights the roles of vascular insufficiency, mitochondrial dysfunction, excitotoxicity, and immune system dysregulation. The interplay between mechanical stress at the lamina cribrosa and compromised blood supply leads to axonal degeneration and progressive loss of retinal ganglion cells. Additionally, inflammatory responses and oxidative stress exacerbate cellular damage, creating a cycle of neurodegeneration that continues even after IOP is controlled. By dissecting these pathophysiological mechanisms, we gain insight into potential neuroprotective strategies that may halt or slow disease progression.

The second section, "Types of Glaucoma: Open-Angle vs. Angle-Closure," provides a detailed comparison of the two major clinical subtypes of glaucoma. Primary open-angle glaucoma (POAG) is the most prevalent form, characterized by a gradual increase in IOP due to impaired aqueous humor outflow through the trabecular meshwork. In contrast, primary angle-closure glaucoma (PACG) involves a structural narrowing of the anterior chamber angle, leading to intermittent or sustained IOP elevation. This section examines the distinct anatomical and physiological differences between these subtypes, highlighting risk factors, diagnostic features, and treatment approaches tailored to each form. Furthermore, it discusses secondary forms of glaucoma, which arise from systemic diseases, trauma, or medication-induced changes in ocular physiology, further complicating disease management.

The third section, "Genetic and Environmental Risk Factors," delves into the hereditary and external influences that contribute to glaucoma susceptibility. Genetic predisposition plays a significant role, with multiple genes, including MYOC, OPTN, and TBK1, linked to glaucoma development. Advances in genome-wide

DOI: 10.1201/9781003646693-3

association studies (GWAS) have identified several risk loci associated with IOP regulation and optic nerve resilience. However, environmental factors such as age, ethnicity, lifestyle, systemic diseases, and medication use also modulate disease onset and progression. This section explores the relationship between genetic and environmental components, emphasizing the need for personalized risk assessment and early intervention strategies.

By examining the pathophysiological underpinnings of glaucoma, this chapter provides a comprehensive understanding of disease mechanisms, classifications, and risk factors. This knowledge not only informs clinical decision-making but also paves the way for future research aimed at developing innovative treatment modalities and improving patient care.

SECTION I—MECHANISMS OF OPTIC NERVE DAMAGE

Glaucomatous optic neuropathy represents a complex pathological cascade that ultimately leads to the progressive degeneration of retinal ganglion cells (RGCs) and their axons. While elevated intraocular pressure (IOP) has traditionally been considered the primary risk factor, research over the past two decades has revealed a multidimensional pathophysiology involving several interconnected mechanisms. This section examines the key pathological processes that contribute to optic nerve damage in glaucoma.

Figure 3.1 illustrates the difference between a healthy eye and an eye with glaucoma. Elevated IOP remains the most established and modifiable risk factor for

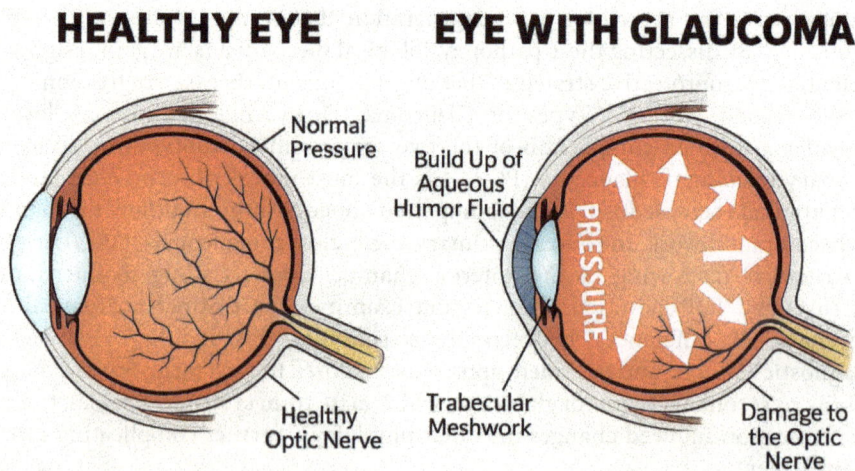

HEALTHY EYE   **EYE WITH GLAUCOMA**

Normal Pressure
Healthy Optic Nerve
Build Up of Aqueous Humor Fluid
PRESSURE
Trabecular Meshwork
Damage to the Optic Nerve

Figure 3.1 Healthy vs. glaucomatous eye.

glaucomatous damage. The mechanical theory posits that increased pressure within the eye creates biomechanical stress at the lamina cribrosa, a specialized structure through which the optic nerve fibers exit the eye. This pressure-induced stress leads to several detrimental effects.

The lamina cribrosa undergoes remodeling and posterior displacement, creating a mechanical strain on the axons passing through it. This strain disrupts axonal transport, preventing the movement of essential neurotrophic factors, mitochondria, and other cellular components necessary for RGC survival. The compromised axoplasmic flow results in a state of neurotrophic deprivation, particularly affecting brain-derived neurotrophic factor (BDNF) and nerve growth factor (NGF), which are critical for maintaining neuronal health and function. The mechanical compression also directly damages axonal microtubules and microfilaments, further compromising structural integrity and cellular transport mechanisms. Over time, this pressure-induced damage initiates a series of events that culminate in axonal degeneration and subsequent RGC apoptosis. The pattern of damage typically follows a characteristic sequence, with preferential loss of larger diameter axons in the superior and inferior regions of the optic nerve, corresponding to the arcuate defects seen in visual field testing.

However, the mechanical theory alone cannot fully explain the pathophysiology of glaucoma. Approximately one-third of glaucoma patients have normal-tension glaucoma, where optic nerve damage occurs despite IOP within the statistically normal range. Additionally, some patients with ocular hypertension never develop glaucomatous damage despite sustained elevated pressures. These observations have led to the exploration of additional factors contributing to glaucomatous optic neuropathy.

The vascular theory proposes that insufficient blood supply to the optic nerve head plays a critical role in glaucomatous damage. Several mechanisms contribute to this vascular compromise: Autoregulatory dysfunction impairs the eye's ability to maintain consistent blood flow despite fluctuations in IOP or systemic blood pressure. This dysfunction is particularly pronounced in patients with primary open-angle glaucoma and normal-tension glaucoma, who often exhibit impaired endothelium-dependent vasodilation. Structural changes in the microcirculation of the optic nerve head, including capillary dropout and basement membrane thickening, further compromise perfusion. Vasospasm, more prevalent in patients with migraine and Raynaud's phenomenon, causes transient ischemic episodes that may contribute to cumulative damage over time. The resulting ischemia-reperfusion injury generates reactive oxygen species (ROS) that damage cellular components and trigger inflammatory responses. The optic nerve head is particularly vulnerable to ischemic damage due to its unique anatomical and vascular characteristics, with the prelaminar and laminar regions receiving blood supply from different sources. Interestingly, systemic vascular disorders such as hypertension, hypotension (particularly nocturnal dips), diabetes, and atherosclerosis are associated with increased glaucoma risk, supporting the vascular theory of pathogenesis.

Glutamate, the primary excitatory neurotransmitter in the retina, can become neurotoxic when present in excessive concentrations. In glaucoma, several processes contribute to glutamate-mediated excitotoxicity: Mechanical stress and ischemia lead to abnormal glutamate release from damaged cells. Simultaneously, dysfunction of glutamate transporters in Müller cells and astrocytes reduces glutamate clearance from the extracellular space. The resulting elevation in extracellular glutamate overstimulates N-methyl-D-aspartate (NMDA) receptors on RGCs. This excessive NMDA receptor activation triggers a massive influx of calcium ions, activating calcium-dependent enzymes such as calpains and phospholipases that degrade cellular structures. Additionally, calcium overload disrupts mitochondrial function, leading to energy depletion and increased ROS production. The excitotoxic cascade ultimately converges on apoptotic pathways, activating caspases and other pro-apoptotic proteins. Studies have found elevated glutamate levels in the vitreous of glaucoma patients, and experimental models demonstrate that excessive glutamate exposure reproduces patterns of damage similar to those seen in glaucoma.

The retina and optic nerve have high metabolic demands and are particularly susceptible to oxidative damage. Several factors contribute to oxidative stress in glaucoma: Mitochondrial dysfunction, observed in both experimental models and clinical studies of glaucoma, leads to decreased ATP production and increased ROS generation. The high energy requirements of unmyelinated RGC axons in the prelaminar region make them especially vulnerable to energy deficits. Impaired antioxidant defense mechanisms further exacerbate oxidative damage. Reduced levels of glutathione, superoxide dismutase, and other antioxidant enzymes have been reported in glaucoma patients. Oxidative stress damages cellular components including proteins, lipids, and DNA, particularly mitochondrial DNA which lacks robust repair mechanisms. This creates a vicious cycle where mitochondrial damage leads to further ROS production. The accumulation of advanced glycation end products (AGEs) and advanced lipoxidation end products (ALEs) contributes to extracellular matrix remodeling and further cellular damage. These modifications also trigger inflammatory responses, linking oxidative stress to neuroinflammation.

Emerging evidence suggests that inflammatory processes contribute significantly to glaucomatous damage: Activated astrocytes and microglia release pro-inflammatory cytokines, including tumor necrosis factor-alpha (TNF-α), interleukin-1β (IL-1β), and interleukin-6 (IL-6). These cytokines promote further microglial activation, creating a self-perpetuating inflammatory cycle. Complement activation, particularly involving the classical pathway, has been observed in glaucomatous retinas. Complement components can directly damage neuronal membranes through the formation of the membrane attack complex. Autoimmune mechanisms may also play a role, with evidence of circulating autoantibodies against retinal antigens such as heat shock proteins (HSPs) and retinal S-antigen in some glaucoma patients. These autoantibodies potentially cross-react with retinal antigens following breakdown of the blood–retina barrier.

The inflammatory environment promotes the expression of matrix metall-oproteinases (MMPs) that remodel the extracellular matrix, potentially altering tissue biomechanics and exacerbating mechanical strain.

Neurotrophic factors, including BDNF, NGF, and ciliary neurotrophic factor (CNTF), are essential for RGC survival and function. In glaucoma, several mechanisms contribute to neurotrophic factor deprivation: Disrupted retrograde axonal transport prevents the delivery of target-derived neurotrophic factors from the brain to RGC bodies. Mechanical compression at the lamina cribrosa and energy deficits from mitochondrial dysfunction contribute to this transport failure. Altered expression of neurotrophic factors and their receptors has been observed in glaucomatous eyes. For example, TrkB receptor expression decreases in response to elevated IOP, reducing RGC responsiveness to available BDNF. Neurotrophic factor deprivation activates pro-apoptotic pathways, including the JNK/c-Jun pathway and the p75NTR-mediated apoptotic cascade. This ultimately leads to caspase activation and programmed cell death.

Regardless of the initiating factors, the pathways described previously ultimately converge on apoptosis as the predominant mode of RGC death in glaucoma: The intrinsic (mitochondrial) pathway involves the release of cytochrome c and other pro-apoptotic factors from mitochondria, leading to the formation of the apoptosome and activation of caspase-9 and caspase–3. Bcl-2 family proteins, particularly the balance between pro-apoptotic (Bax, Bad) and anti-apoptotic (Bcl-2, Bcl-xL) members, regulate this pathway. The extrinsic pathway, activated by inflammatory cytokines such as TNF-α binding to death receptors, leads to the formation of the death-inducing signaling complex (DISC) and activation of caspase-8 and caspase-3.

Caspase-independent mechanisms, including the release of apoptosis-inducing factor (AIF) and endonuclease G from mitochondria, contribute to DNA fragmentation and apoptotic cell death.

Evidence suggests that apoptosis may begin in the dendrites of RGCs and progress retrograde to the cell body, a process termed "compartmentalized self-destruction." This progressive degeneration may explain the long preclinical phase observed in many glaucoma patients.

The pathophysiology of glaucomatous optic neuropathy represents a complex interplay of mechanical, vascular, metabolic, inflammatory, and apoptotic mechanisms. Rather than operating in isolation, these pathways interact and reinforce each other, creating a cascade of damage that ultimately leads to RGC death and irreversible vision loss. Understanding these mechanisms has significant implications for therapeutic approaches, suggesting that comprehensive glaucoma management should extend beyond IOP control to include neuroprotective strategies targeting these various pathways. Furthermore, the diversity of mechanisms involved explains the clinical heterogeneity observed in glaucoma, with different patients exhibiting varying susceptibility to specific pathophysiological processes based on their genetic background and environmental exposures.

SECTION 2—TYPES OF GLAUCOMA: OPEN-ANGLE VS. ANGLE-CLOSURE

Glaucoma encompasses a diverse group of optic neuropathies with distinct etiologies, pathophysiological mechanisms, clinical presentations, and treatment approaches. While the previous section explored the common pathways of optic nerve damage, this section examines the major classifications of glaucoma with particular emphasis on the two predominant categories: open-angle and angle-closure glaucoma. Understanding these distinctions is essential for accurate diagnosis, risk assessment, and implementation of appropriate therapeutic strategies. The classification of glaucoma primarily relies on the status of the anterior chamber angle, the anatomical junction between the peripheral cornea and the iris. This angle houses the trabecular meshwork, the primary pathway for aqueous humor outflow. Gonioscopic examination of this region reveals critical structures including the iris root, ciliary body band, scleral spur, and trabecular meshwork, assessment of which forms the basis for distinguishing between open-angle and angle-closure glaucoma.

In open-angle glaucoma, the angle structures are visible on gonioscopic examination, and the peripheral iris does not obstruct the trabecular meshwork. In contrast, angle-closure glaucoma is characterized by apposition between the peripheral iris and the trabecular meshwork, resulting in partial or complete obstruction of the angle. This fundamental anatomical distinction underlies the divergent pathophysiological mechanisms, clinical presentations, and management approaches for these two major categories.

Primary Open-Angle Glaucoma (POAG)

Primary open-angle glaucoma represents the most prevalent form of glaucoma worldwide, accounting for approximately 74% of all glaucoma cases. It is characterized by progressive optic neuropathy with corresponding visual field defects, open anterior chamber angles, and typically, but not invariably, elevated intraocular pressure. The primary pathophysiological mechanism in POAG involves increased resistance to aqueous outflow through the trabecular meshwork and Schlemm's canal. Several factors contribute to this impaired outflow: Histopathological studies reveal accumulation of extracellular matrix material in the juxtacanalicular region of the trabecular meshwork, particularly glycosaminoglycans and cross-linked collagen. This accumulation reduces the effective filtration area and increases outflow resistance. Trabecular meshwork cells demonstrate age-related and oxidative stress-induced changes, including decreased cellularity, altered cytoskeletal organization, and impaired phagocytic capacity. These cellular changes compromise the meshwork's ability to maintain normal aqueous outflow channels. Dysregulation of matrix metalloproteinases (MMPs) and their tissue inhibitors disrupts the normal balance of extracellular matrix turnover, favoring accumulation of matrix components that obstruct outflow pathways. Increased stiffness of the trabecular meshwork and Schlemm's canal reduces their distensibility in response to pressure changes, further compromising outflow facility. The role of the conventional outflow pathway (trabecular meshwork and Schlemm's canal) versus the unconventional pathway (uveoscleral outflow) in the pathogenesis of POAG continues to be an area of active research, with therapeutic implications for selectively targeting these outflow routes.

POAG typically presents as a bilateral, asymmetric, chronic, and slowly progressive disease. Its insidious nature often leads to delayed diagnosis, with many patients remaining asymptomatic until significant optic nerve damage and visual field loss have occurred. Key diagnostic features are as follows: Open anterior chamber angles on gonioscopic examination, with normal anatomical appearance of angle structures. Characteristic optic nerve head changes, including progressive thinning of the neuroretinal rim, vertical elongation of the optic cup, notching of the rim, and peripapillary retinal nerve fiber layer defects. Corresponding visual field defects, typically beginning as paracentral scotomas or nasal steps, and progressing to arcuate defects and eventually central vision loss in advanced disease.

Elevated IOP (>21 mmHg) is present in many but not all cases, highlighting the importance of considering POAG in patients with normal IOP who demonstrate progressive optic neuropathy. Advanced diagnostic technologies, including optical coherence tomography (OCT), confocal scanning laser ophthalmoscopy, and scanning laser polarimetry, provide quantitative assessment of structural changes often preceding detectable functional deficits on perimetry.

Normal-Tension Glaucoma (NTG)

Next, normal-tension glaucoma represents a significant subset of POAG, characterized by glaucomatous optic neuropathy and visual field defects despite IOP consistently within the statistically normal range (≤21 mmHg). The pathophysiology of NTG likely involves increased susceptibility of the optic nerve to normal pressure levels due to the following: Vascular dysregulation, with evidence of impaired autoregulation, vasospasm, and nocturnal hypotension contributing to optic nerve head ischemia. Biomechanical vulnerability, with thinner lamina cribrosa and altered scleral properties increasing susceptibility to pressure-induced damage even at normal IOP levels. Genetic factors, including certain polymorphisms associated with increased NTG risk, such as those in the optineurin (OPTN) and TANK binding kinase 1 (TBK1) genes. NTG patients typically present with deeper and more localized optic disc cupping and visual field defects that may be more likely to involve the central visual field compared to high-pressure POAG. Despite these differences, IOP reduction remains a cornerstone of NTG management, with studies demonstrating that even modest pressure reductions can slow disease progression.

Primary Angle-Closure Glaucoma (PACG)

Primary angle-closure glaucoma, though less prevalent globally than POAG, carries a higher risk of bilateral blindness and accounts for a significant proportion of glaucoma cases, particularly in Asian populations. PACG represents a spectrum of disease from the initial anatomical predisposition (primary angle-closure suspect) to established glaucomatous optic neuropathy (primary angle-closure glaucoma). The fundamental pathophysiological mechanism in PACG involves appositional or synechial closure of the anterior chamber angle, obstructing aqueous outflow through the trabecular meshwork. Several anatomical predisposing factors contribute to angle closure: Shallow anterior chamber depth, typically due to a more anteriorly positioned lens or smaller overall anterior segment dimensions. Increased lens thickness and anterior positioning is often age related, which reduces the space between the iris and lens (iridolenticular contact). Shorter axial length and hyperopic refractive error, creating a crowded anterior segment with predisposition to angle closure. Plateau iris configuration, characterized by an anteriorly positioned ciliary body that pushes the peripheral iris forward despite a normal central anterior chamber depth.

These anatomical factors can lead to various mechanisms of angle closure: Pupillary block, the most common mechanism, occurs when aqueous humor cannot flow freely from the posterior chamber to the anterior chamber due to excessive apposition between the iris and lens. This creates a pressure gradient that forces the peripheral iris anteriorly, closing the angle. Non-pupillary block mechanisms include plateau iris syndrome, lens-induced angle closure, and ciliary block (malignant) glaucoma, each with distinct pathophysiological features requiring specific management approaches.

PACG represents a disease spectrum with several distinct clinical entities: Primary angle-closure suspect (PACS) refers to anatomically narrow angles without elevated IOP or peripheral anterior synechiae (PAS). These patients have the potential for angle closure but have not yet developed the condition. Primary angle closure (PAC) involves an occludable angle with evidence of trabecular obstruction, such as elevated IOP or PAS, but without optic nerve damage or visual field defects. Primary angle-closure glaucoma (PACG) represents the full syndrome with angle closure, elevated IOP, and glaucomatous optic neuropathy with corresponding visual field loss.

The clinical presentation varies considerably across this spectrum: Acute angle-closure represents the most dramatic presentation, characterized by sudden IOP elevation (often >50 mmHg) with symptoms including severe ocular pain, headache, nausea, vomiting, and blurred vision. Clinical signs include conjunctival injection, corneal edema, mid-dilated unreactive pupil, and shallow anterior chamber. This constitutes an ophthalmological emergency requiring immediate intervention to prevent irreversible vision loss.

Subacute (intermittent) angle-closure presents with recurrent episodes of angle closure with spontaneous resolution, often triggered by conditions promoting pupillary dilation such as dim lighting or emotional stress. Symptoms include transient blurring of vision, halos around lights, and mild ocular discomfort.

Chronic angle-closure develops insidiously with gradual synechial closure of the angle, often asymptomatic until advanced stages similar to POAG. Careful gonioscopic examination is essential to distinguish chronic PACG from POAG, as the management approaches differ significantly.

Secondary Glaucomas

Secondary glaucomas encompass a diverse group of disorders where glaucomatous optic neuropathy results from identifiable ocular or systemic conditions. These forms may present with either open or closed angles, with mechanisms often overlapping those of primary glaucomas but with distinct etiologies.

Secondary Open-Angle Glaucomas

Pseudoexfoliation glaucoma results from deposition of fibrillar material in the anterior segment, including the trabecular meshwork, leading to increased outflow resistance. It is characterized by more aggressive IOP elevation and faster progression than POAG. Pigmentary glaucoma occurs when pigment from the iris epithelium detaches and obstructs the trabecular meshwork, typically affecting young myopic males. Posterior iris bowing and iris-zonule contact contribute to pigment dispersion. Inflammatory (uveitic) glaucoma develops from trabecular obstruction by inflammatory cells and debris, trabeculitis, or steroid-induced elevation of IOP in the context of intraocular inflammation.

Lens-related open-angle glaucoma includes phacolytic glaucoma from leakage of lens proteins in mature cataracts and lens particle glaucoma following cataract surgery or trauma with retained lens material. Steroid-induced glaucoma results from increased resistance to aqueous outflow following topical or systemic corticosteroid administration, with substantial individual variability in susceptibility.

Secondary Angle-Closure Glaucomas

Neovascular glaucoma develops from fibrovascular membrane formation over the angle structures in response to retinal ischemia, most commonly from diabetic retinopathy or central retinal vein occlusion. Iridocorneal endothelial (ICE) syndrome encompasses a spectrum of disorders with abnormal corneal endothelium proliferating across the angle and iris, forming peripheral anterior synechiae and secondary angle closure. Aqueous misdirection (malignant glaucoma) involves posterior misdirection of aqueous humor into or behind the vitreous, creating a vicious cycle of increasing vitreous pressure and progressive shallowing of the anterior chamber.

Developmental Glaucomas

Developmental glaucomas encompass a range of disorders with onset from birth to early adulthood, resulting from abnormal development of the anterior segment structures. These include: Primary congenital glaucoma, resulting from isolated trabeculodysgenesis with impaired aqueous outflow. Juvenile open-angle glaucoma, with onset between 5 and 35 years of age, often with more aggressive progression than adult-onset POAG. Glaucoma associated with systemic disorders or ocular anomalies, including Axenfeld–Rieger syndrome, Peters anomaly, aniridia, and Sturge–Weber syndrome.

The classification of glaucoma into open-angle and angle-closure categories provides a fundamental framework for understanding the diverse pathophysiological mechanisms, clinical presentations, and therapeutic approaches for this complex disease. While POAG and PACG represent the predominant categories, the spectrum of glaucomatous disorders extends to numerous secondary and developmental forms, each with unique challenges for diagnosis and management. The evolution of advanced imaging technologies, genetic testing, and molecular biomarkers continues to refine our classification systems, moving toward more personalized approaches to glaucoma diagnosis and treatment. Accurate classification remains the cornerstone of effective glaucoma management, guiding clinicians in selecting appropriate interventions to preserve vision and maintain quality of life for affected individuals.

Although glaucoma represents a diverse group of diseases, anatomical variations within the eye are key determinants of different glaucoma subtypes. Table 3.1 offers a comparative summary of major glaucoma types, outlining their defining anatomical abnormalities, typical intraocular pressure patterns, and distinctive clinical characteristics essential for accurate diagnosis and treatment planning.

Table 3.1 Types of Glaucoma and Associated Anatomical Features

Glaucoma Type	Primary Anatomical Abnormality	Typical IOP Findings	Notes
Primary Open-Angle Glaucoma (POAG)	Dysfunctional trabecular meshwork	Elevated	Chronic, asymptomatic
Primary Angle-Closure Glaucoma (PACG)	Narrow/closed anterior chamber angle	Sudden, very high	Ocular emergency
Normal-Tension Glaucoma (NTG)	Optic nerve vulnerability despite normal IOP	Normal	Vascular factors key
Secondary Glaucomas	Varies: Pigment, inflammation, trauma	Variable	Must treat underlying cause

SECTION 3—GENETIC AND ENVIRONMENTAL RISK FACTORS

Understanding the complex interplay between genetic predisposition and environmental influences is fundamental to comprehending glaucoma's etiology, progression, and management. While elevated intraocular pressure remains the primary modifiable risk factor, a multitude of genetic and environmental elements contribute to individual susceptibility and disease manifestation. Recent advances in genomic technologies have significantly expanded our knowledge of the hereditary aspects of glaucoma, while epidemiological studies continue to identify crucial environmental and demographic factors that modulate disease risk. This section explores these diverse risk factors and their implications for screening, diagnosis, and personalized treatment approaches.

The hereditary nature of glaucoma has been recognized since the early 20th century, with family history consistently emerging as a significant risk factor across multiple epidemiological studies. First-degree relatives of glaucoma patients demonstrate a 9–10-fold increased risk compared to the general population, with the strength of familial association varying among different glaucoma subtypes. The genetic architecture of glaucoma is notably heterogeneous, encompassing monogenic forms with Mendelian inheritance patterns as well as more common complex forms influenced by multiple genetic variants in conjunction with environmental factors.

Monogenic forms of glaucoma, though relatively rare, have provided invaluable insights into the molecular pathways underlying the disease. Primary congenital glaucoma, for instance, is predominantly associated with mutations in the CYP1B1 gene, which encodes a cytochrome P450 enzyme involved in ocular development and metabolism of endogenous compounds. These mutations disrupt trabecular meshwork development, resulting in impaired aqueous outflow and early-onset glaucoma. Similarly, juvenile-onset open-angle glaucoma often demonstrates autosomal dominant inheritance linked to mutations in the MYOC gene, which encodes myocilin, a protein expressed in the trabecular meshwork. Pathogenic MYOC mutations lead to protein misfolding and accumulation in trabecular meshwork cells, triggering endoplasmic reticulum stress and ultimately cellular dysfunction and death. This mechanism progressively compromises aqueous outflow facility, resulting in elevated IOP and subsequent optic nerve damage.

Beyond these monogenic forms, several genes have been implicated in adult-onset primary open-angle glaucoma with varying penetrance and expressivity. The optineurin (OPTN) gene, mutations in which were initially associated with normal-tension glaucoma, encodes a protein involved in cellular processes including vesicle trafficking, maintenance of the Golgi apparatus, and autophagy. OPTN also plays a role in TNF-α signaling and NF-κB regulation, linking it to neuroinflammatory processes relevant to glaucomatous optic neuropathy. Similarly, mutations in the TANK binding kinase 1 (TBK1) gene, which functions in the same pathway as OPTN, have been identified in normal-tension glaucoma families, further highlighting the importance of these molecular pathways in glaucoma pathogenesis.

Genome-wide association studies (GWAS) have revolutionized our understanding of the genetic landscape of glaucoma, revealing numerous common genetic variants with modest individual effects that collectively contribute substantially to disease risk. These studies have identified multiple loci associated with POAG, including TMCO1, CAV1/CAV2, ABCA1, AFAP1, GMDS, PMM2, TGFBR3, and FNDC3B, among others. Many of these genes participate in pathways relevant to glaucoma pathogenesis, including extracellular matrix remodeling, cytoskeletal organization, mitochondrial function, and cellular stress responses. Notably, several genetic loci, such as those near the genes CDKN2B-AS1 and SIX1/SIX6, associate more strongly with features of optic nerve structure and glaucomatous damage rather than with IOP, suggesting distinct genetic contributions to the pressure-independent aspects of glaucomatous optic neuropathy.

The genetic architecture of primary angle-closure glaucoma appears similarly complex but with distinct molecular underpinnings. GWAS studies in Asian populations, where PACG is more prevalent, have identified susceptibility loci including PLEKHA7, COL11A1, PCMTD1-ST18, EPDR1, and GLIS3. Many of these genes influence anterior segment anatomy, potentially contributing to the shallower anterior chambers and narrower angles characteristic of PACG predisposition. These genetic insights align with the anatomical basis of angle-closure glaucoma and suggest that distinct molecular pathways contribute to different glaucoma subtypes.

Genetic risk assessment for glaucoma continues to evolve from single-gene testing toward polygenic risk scores that integrate the effects of multiple genetic variants. These polygenic approaches have demonstrated increasing ability to identify individuals at elevated risk for developing glaucoma and may eventually guide personalized screening and preventive interventions. Pharmacogenomics, examining how genetic variation influences response to glaucoma medications, represents another promising frontier, potentially enabling tailored therapy based on individual genetic profiles. For instance, certain polymorphisms in the beta-adrenergic receptor genes have been associated with variable responsiveness to beta-blocker medications, while variations in prostaglandin pathway genes may influence response to prostaglandin analog therapies.

While genetic predisposition significantly influences glaucoma susceptibility, numerous environmental and demographic factors modulate disease risk, progression, and treatment outcomes. These factors span demographic characteristics, systemic medical conditions, lifestyle elements, and medication exposures, many of which interact with genetic risk factors through complex gene–environment interactions.

Age represents perhaps the most established demographic risk factor for glaucoma, particularly for POAG, with prevalence increasing dramatically after age 40. This age-associated risk reflects cumulative cellular and tissue changes including trabecular meshwork dysfunction, decreased outflow facility, increased lens thickness, and reduced optic nerve resilience. The aging optic nerve demonstrates decreased axonal transport capacity, mitochondrial dysfunction, and impaired ability to withstand insults, creating increased vulnerability to glaucomatous damage. These age-related changes may explain why older individuals often demonstrate glaucomatous progression despite apparently well-controlled IOP, necessitating more aggressive target pressures in advanced age.

Ethnicity constitutes another significant demographic factor influencing glaucoma risk and phenotype. Individuals of African descent demonstrate substantially higher POAG prevalence, earlier disease onset, more rapid progression, and increased risk of blindness compared to European-derived populations. Anatomical differences in the optic nerve head, including larger disc area and deeper cupping, may contribute to this increased susceptibility, along with differences in trabecular meshwork structure and function. Conversely, PACG demonstrates higher prevalence in East Asian populations, attributed to anatomical variations including shallower anterior chambers, thicker lenses, and smaller corneal diameters. These ethnic differences highlight the importance of culturally sensitive screening programs and community-specific interventions, particularly in regions with limited healthcare access where glaucoma often remains undiagnosed until advanced stages.

Myopia, particularly moderate to high myopia, associates with increased POAG risk through several potential mechanisms. The elongated axial length in myopic eyes creates structural changes at the optic nerve head, including thinning of the lamina cribrosa and sclera, potentially increasing vulnerability to pressure-induced damage. Additionally, myopic eyes may demonstrate altered biomechanical properties that influence strain distribution within the optic nerve tissues. Interestingly, while myopia increases POAG risk, it appears protective against PACG due to the associated deeper anterior chambers and wider angle configurations. The growing global prevalence of myopia, particularly in East Asian populations, may influence future patterns of glaucoma distribution and necessitate targeted screening approaches for high-risk myopic individuals.

Numerous systemic medical conditions influence glaucoma risk and progression. Vascular factors feature prominently among these associations, with systemic hypertension demonstrating a complex relationship with glaucoma risk. While chronic hypertension may initially protect against glaucomatous damage by maintaining adequate optic nerve perfusion despite elevated IOP, long-standing hypertension ultimately promotes vascular sclerosis and endothelial dysfunction, compromising autoregulatory capacity and increasing susceptibility to optic nerve ischemia. Conversely, systemic hypotension, particularly nocturnal dips in blood pressure, may reduce optic nerve perfusion below critical thresholds, especially in patients with impaired autoregulation. This phenomenon, termed "nocturnal dipping," has been associated with progressive visual field loss despite apparently controlled IOP, emphasizing the importance of 24-hour blood pressure monitoring in selected patients with progressive normal-tension glaucoma.

Diabetes mellitus influences glaucoma risk through multiple mechanisms. Hyperglycemia induces trabecular meshwork damage through advanced glycation end product formation, oxidative stress, and mitochondrial dysfunction, potentially increasing outflow resistance and IOP. Diabetic microvascular disease compromises optic nerve head perfusion and may impair neurotrophic factor delivery to retinal ganglion cells. Additionally, diabetes-associated autonomic dysfunction may affect ocular blood flow regulation, creating increased vulnerability to pressure fluctuations. While epidemiological studies show somewhat inconsistent associations between diabetes and glaucoma risk, the biological plausibility of this relationship warrants careful monitoring of diabetic patients for glaucomatous changes.

Sleep apnea has emerged as an increasingly recognized risk factor for glaucoma, particularly normal-tension variants. The recurrent nocturnal hypoxia characteristic of obstructive sleep apnea creates oxidative stress, impairs vascular endothelial function, and promotes inflammation, potentially contributing to optic nerve vulnerability. Episodes of apnea also associate with transient IOP elevations and blood pressure fluctuations that may further compromise optic nerve health. Growing evidence suggests that continuous positive airway pressure therapy for sleep apnea may help stabilize glaucomatous progression in affected individuals, highlighting the importance of identifying and addressing this modifiable risk factor.

Lifestyle factors including exercise, dietary patterns, and substance use may influence glaucoma risk and progression. Regular aerobic exercise typically reduces IOP through multiple mechanisms including decreased sympathetic tone, enhanced nitric oxide-mediated vasodilation, and potentially improved trabecular outflow facility. However, certain exercise modalities, particularly those involving Valsalva maneuvers or inverted positions, may transiently increase IOP and should be approached cautiously in glaucoma patients. Dietary factors with potential influence on glaucoma risk include antioxidant intake, omega-3 fatty acid consumption, and caffeine exposure, although definitive evidence for dietary interventions remains limited. Tobacco use consistently emerges as a risk factor for glaucoma, likely through promotion of oxidative stress, vascular dysfunction, and inflammation, providing additional rationale for smoking cessation counseling in glaucoma patients.

Medication exposure represents important modifiable risk factors for glaucoma, with corticosteroids being the most established pharmacological influence. Approximately 30–40% of the general population demonstrates ocular hypertensive responses to topical corticosteroids, with higher susceptibility among POAG patients and their first-degree relatives. This steroid response involves upregulation of extracellular matrix components in the trabecular meshwork, decreased phagocytic capacity, and cytoskeletal reorganization, collectively impairing aqueous outflow. Corticosteroid-induced glaucoma can develop from topical, periocular, intravitreal, inhaled, or even high-dose systemic corticosteroid exposure, necessitating careful IOP monitoring in exposed individuals, particularly those with existing glaucoma risk factors.

The interface between genetic predisposition and environmental exposures represents an emerging frontier in glaucoma research. Several studies suggest that genetic variants may modify the influence of environmental factors on glaucoma risk and progression. For instance, certain polymorphisms in nitric oxide synthase genes appear to modify the association between primary vascular dysregulation and normal-tension glaucoma, potentially explaining why only some patients with vasospastic tendencies develop glaucomatous damage. Similarly, genetic variants involved in trabecular meshwork extracellular matrix metabolism may influence individual susceptibility to steroid-induced ocular hypertension, creating opportunities for pharmacogenomic approaches to predict and prevent this adverse effect.

The concept of epigenetics—heritable changes in gene expression that do not involve alterations in DNA sequence—provides another framework for understanding gene–environment interactions in glaucoma. Environmental factors including oxidative stress, hypoxia, and inflammation can induce epigenetic modifications such as DNA methylation, histone modifications, and microRNA expression changes that alter the expression of genes relevant to glaucoma pathogenesis. These epigenetic mechanisms may partially explain the age-related increases in glaucoma risk, as well as the influence of environmental exposures on disease susceptibility and progression. Epigenetic markers represent potential biomarkers for glaucoma risk and may eventually provide targets for novel therapeutic approaches.

The expanding knowledge of genetic and environmental risk factors for glaucoma has profound implications for clinical practice and research. Risk stratification integrating genetic, demographic, and medical factors can guide screening frequency and intensity, potentially enabling earlier detection in high-risk individuals. Genetic testing, particularly for highly penetrant mutations in monogenic forms of glaucoma, allows identification of at-risk family members and may guide reproductive decision-making. As polygenic risk scores continue to improve in predictive capacity, they may eventually guide population-level screening programs and facilitate more personalized treatment approaches.

Modifiable risk factors provide opportunities for preventive interventions beyond IOP control. Optimal management of systemic conditions including hypertension, diabetes, and sleep apnea may help preserve optic nerve health. Lifestyle modifications including regular exercise, smoking cessation, and potentially dietary adjustments represent low-risk interventions that may complement traditional glaucoma therapies. Careful medication reviews to minimize exposure to IOP-elevating drugs, particularly corticosteroids, represent another avenue for risk modification.

Future research directions include expanded genomic studies in diverse populations to identify additional risk loci and clarify population-specific genetic factors. Integration of genetic data with detailed phenotypic characterization may reveal distinct glaucoma endophenotypes with specific genetic and environmental risk profiles, potentially enabling more targeted therapeutic approaches. Longitudinal studies assessing how gene–environment interactions influence disease progression will provide insights into the dynamics of glaucomatous damage and may identify new windows for therapeutic intervention.

The ultimate goal of this research lies in translating these insights into personalized prevention and treatment strategies. By understanding the specific genetic, anatomical, vascular, and environmental factors contributing to each patient's glaucoma risk, clinicians may eventually tailor screening intervals, target pressures, medication choices, and surgical approaches to the individual's unique risk profile. This precision medicine approach represents the frontier of glaucoma management, promising improved outcomes through interventions specifically matched to each patient's underlying disease mechanisms rather than generic approaches based solely on IOP measurements and disease staging.

CHAPTER 4
DIAGNOSIS OF
GLAUCOMA

The accurate and timely diagnosis of glaucoma represents one of the most significant challenges in ophthalmic practice. As a progressive optic neuropathy that is often asymptomatic until advanced stages, glaucoma requires vigilant screening, comprehensive assessment, and precise diagnostic techniques to identify the disease before irreversible vision loss occurs. The diagnostic approach to glaucoma has evolved considerably over the past several decades, transitioning from a singular focus on intraocular pressure to a more complex evaluation of structural and functional parameters that collectively define the disease.

The diagnostic paradigm for glaucoma incorporates three essential components: structural assessment of the optic nerve head and retinal nerve fiber layer, functional evaluation of visual fields, and measurement of intraocular pressure in the context of anterior segment examination. This integrated approach acknowledges the complex nature of glaucoma as a disease with diverse presentations, subtypes, and progression patterns, necessitating a customized diagnostic strategy for each patient. Furthermore, the recognition of glaucoma as a continuum—from early pre-perimetric stages to advanced disease—has highlighted the importance of detecting subtle changes that may precede conventional clinical manifestations.

Technological advancements have revolutionized glaucoma diagnostics, providing unprecedented ability to detect and quantify structural and functional abnormalities with increasing sensitivity and specificity. From sophisticated imaging modalities that visualize microscopic changes in the optic nerve head architecture to artificial intelligence algorithms that identify patterns imperceptible to the human eye, these innovations have expanded our capacity to diagnose glaucoma at earlier stages and monitor progression with greater precision. However, the proliferation of diagnostic technologies also presents challenges in interpretation, clinical integration, and cost-effectiveness, requiring judicious application in clinical practice.

Despite these technological advances, the cornerstone of glaucoma diagnosis remains the comprehensive clinical examination conducted by an experienced clinician. The synthesis of patient history, risk factor assessment, slit-lamp biomicroscopy, gonioscopy, and ophthalmoscopy provides the essential framework for interpreting specialized tests and contextualizing their results. Moreover, the differentiation of glaucoma from other optic neuropathies and conditions that mimic glaucomatous damage requires clinical acumen that extends beyond isolated test results or imaging findings.

This chapter explores multiple approaches to glaucoma diagnosis, beginning with fundamental clinical examination techniques that form the foundation of

DOI: 10.1201/9781003646693-4

assessment. It then examines cutting-edge imaging and technological modalities that enhance diagnostic capabilities and concludes with strategies for distinguishing glaucoma from other conditions that may present with similar clinical features. By integrating traditional clinical methods with advanced diagnostic technologies, practitioners can optimize their ability to identify glaucoma at its earliest stages, implement timely interventions, and preserve vision for patients at risk of this potentially blinding disease.

SECTION I—CLINICAL EXAMINATION TECHNIQUES

The clinical examination of a patient with suspected glaucoma encompasses a systematic approach to evaluating the anterior and posterior segments of the eye, with particular attention to structural changes in the optic nerve head, assessment of intraocular pressure, and examination of the anterior chamber angle. These fundamental clinical techniques provide essential diagnostic information that guides further testing and forms the foundation for treatment decisions. While advanced imaging modalities have enhanced our ability to detect and monitor glaucoma, the value of a comprehensive clinical examination performed by an experienced clinician remains paramount in glaucoma diagnosis and management.

Patient History and Risk Factor Assessment

The diagnostic process begins with a thorough history that identifies risk factors for glaucoma development and progression. Key elements include family history of glaucoma, particularly in first-degree relatives, which increases risk by 3–9 fold depending on the subtype of glaucoma. Age is a critical risk factor, with prevalence increasing significantly after age 40 for primary open-angle glaucoma. Racial and ethnic background provides important context, as individuals of African descent have higher risk and earlier onset of POAG, while those of Asian descent have increased prevalence of angle-closure glaucoma.

Medical history should focus on conditions associated with elevated glaucoma risk, including diabetes mellitus, systemic hypertension or hypotension, cardiovascular disease, migraine, Raynaud's phenomenon, and obstructive sleep apnea. A comprehensive medication review is essential to identify agents that may elevate intraocular pressure, most notably corticosteroids in any form (topical, inhaled, oral, or injectable). Prior ocular history, including trauma, inflammation, surgery, or longstanding use of topical medications, may suggest mechanisms for secondary glaucoma.

Symptoms must be carefully evaluated, recognizing that early to moderate glaucoma is typically asymptomatic. However, certain symptoms warrant attention: intermittent blurring of vision or colored halos around lights may indicate intermittent angle closure, while headaches, eye pain, and reduced vision in low light conditions could suggest more advanced disease. Progressive visual field loss typically begins peripherally, often unnoticed by patients until central vision becomes affected in advanced disease.

Visual Acuity and Refraction

Measurement of best-corrected visual acuity serves as a baseline assessment, noting that central visual acuity often remains preserved until late in the disease process. However, contrast sensitivity and visual acuity under low luminance conditions may reveal deficits earlier than standard acuity testing. Refraction is important not only for accurate visual field testing but also because certain refractive errors correlate with glaucoma risk—myopia associates with increased POAG risk, while hyperopia predisposes to angle-closure glaucoma.

Slit-Lamp Biomicroscopy

Slit-lamp examination of the anterior segment provides critical information about potential secondary causes of glaucoma and helps determine the appropriate classification of the disease. Systematic evaluation should include the following:

The cornea, assessed for edema which may indicate elevated IOP, particularly in acute angle closure. Corneal diameter should be noted, as megalocornea may suggest congenital glaucoma, while microcornea may predispose to angle-closure. Corneal thickness measurement (pachymetry) is essential, as central corneal thickness influences tonometric readings and represents an independent risk factor for glaucoma development and progression.

The anterior chamber depth can be estimated using the Van Herick technique, which compares the peripheral anterior chamber depth to corneal thickness. A ratio less than 1:4 suggests a narrow angle requiring gonioscopic evaluation. Signs of previous inflammation, including keratic precipitates, posterior synechiae, or iris transillumination defects, may indicate uveitic or pigmentary mechanisms of secondary glaucoma.

Iris examination may reveal plateau iris configuration, pseudoexfoliation material on the pupillary margin, iris neovascularization suggestive of rubeotic glaucoma, or iris transillumination defects characteristic of pigment dispersion syndrome. Pupillary responses should be assessed, with relative afferent pupillary defect potentially indicating asymmetric glaucomatous damage.

Lens evaluation can identify factors contributing to angle closure, including increased thickness, anterior positioning, intumescence, or dislocation. The presence of pseudoexfoliation material on the anterior lens capsule is pathognomonic for pseudoexfoliative glaucoma, typically appearing as a central disc surrounded by a clear zone and then a peripheral ring of deposition.

Tonometry

Intraocular pressure measurement remains a cornerstone of glaucoma diagnosis and management. Goldmann applanation tonometry continues to be the clinical standard due to its accuracy and reproducibility. However, practitioners must recognize that IOP measurements require adjustment based on central corneal thickness—thinner corneas result in artificially low readings, while thicker corneas lead to artificially high readings. Various correction formulas exist, though no consensus algorithm has been established for clinical use.

A single IOP measurement provides limited information, as intraocular pressure demonstrates diurnal variation of 2–6 mmHg in normal individuals and potentially greater fluctuations in glaucoma patients. When possible, pressure measurements at different times of day provide more comprehensive assessment of IOP control and peak pressures. For selected patients with progressive glaucoma despite apparently controlled office IOP readings, 24-hour pressure monitoring may reveal nocturnal spikes or sustained elevation during periods not captured during office visits.

Alternative tonometry methods include the pneumatonometer (useful for irregular corneas), rebound tonometry (particularly valuable in pediatric populations due to its quick application without anesthesia), and dynamic contour tonometry (which may be less affected by corneal biomechanical properties). Each method has specific advantages and limitations that practitioners must consider when interpreting results.

Gonioscopy

Gonioscopic examination of the anterior chamber angle is essential for proper classification of glaucoma and identification of secondary causes. The technique utilizes special contact lenses containing mirrors or prisms that overcome total internal reflection, allowing visualization of angle structures. Indentation or dynamic gonioscopy helps distinguish between appositional and synechial angle closure and can temporarily open angles closed by appositional mechanisms.

Systematic evaluation assesses the level of iris insertion, the width of the angle recess, and the visibility of structures including the iris root, ciliary body band, scleral spur, trabecular meshwork, and Schwalbe's line. The Shaffer classification system grades angles from 0 (closed) to 4 (wide open) based on the angle between the iris and trabecular meshwork. Alternatively, angle structures visible on gonioscopy can be documented, with visualization of the scleral spur generally indicating an angle not at immediate risk of closure.

Gonioscopy can reveal numerous findings diagnostic of secondary glaucoma, including peripheral anterior synechiae, neovascularization, angle recession, pigmentation of the trabecular meshwork, pseudoexfoliation material, blood in Schlemm's canal, or inflammatory precipitates. The technique remains indispensable despite advances in anterior segment imaging, as it provides dynamic assessment and direct visualization of angle structures.

Figure 4.1 illustrates a gonioscopy image before a gonioscopy-assisted transluminal trabeculotomy (GATT) surgery.

Optic Nerve Head and Retinal Nerve Fiber Layer Examination

Careful evaluation of the optic nerve head constitutes perhaps the most critical component of the clinical examination for glaucoma diagnosis. Stereoscopic assessment through a dilated pupil, using either slit-lamp biomicroscopy with auxiliary lenses (78D, 90D) or direct/indirect ophthalmoscopy, allows appreciation of the three-dimensional structure of the optic disc.

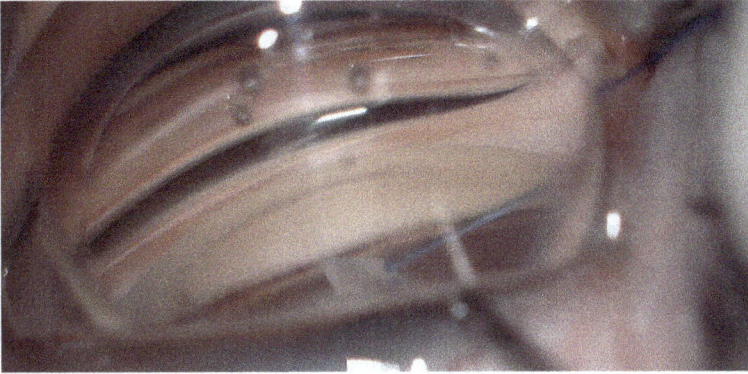

Figure 4.1 A sample gonioscopy image.

Key parameters in optic disc evaluation include the following:

- *Vertical cup-to-disc ratio (CDR)*, recognizing that the average CDR in normal eyes is approximately 0.4, with only 2% of the normal population having a CDR exceeding 0.7. However, CDR must be interpreted in the context of disc size—large discs typically have larger cups, while small discs normally have small or absent cups.
- *Neuroretinal rim assessment* follows the ISNT rule (Inferior > Superior > Nasal > Temporal) for rim thickness in normal eyes. Focal thinning or notching of the rim, particularly superiorly or inferiorly, strongly suggests glaucomatous damage. Progressive rim thinning over time represents a key indicator of ongoing disease activity.
- *Optic disc hemorrhages*, appearing as flame-shaped or splinter hemorrhages at the disc margin, often precede retinal nerve fiber layer defects and visual field loss. These hemorrhages typically resolve within 6–10 weeks but frequently recur and associate with progressive glaucomatous damage at the location of the hemorrhage.
- *Peripapillary atrophy*, particularly zone beta atrophy (adjacent to the disc with visible sclera and large choroidal vessels), correlates with glaucomatous damage and may progress alongside other structural changes. The presence of acquired pits of the optic nerve (APON) strongly indicates glaucomatous damage.
- *Retinal nerve fiber layer assessment* using red-free (green) illumination can reveal wedge-shaped defects or diffuse thinning that often precedes detectable visual field loss. These defects appear as dark areas against the striated pattern of the healthy nerve fiber layer.

Careful documentation of optic nerve findings, through drawings, photographs, or imaging, establishes a baseline for future comparison. Serial evaluation remains crucial for detecting progressive changes characteristic of glaucoma.

Perimetry

While detailed discussion of perimetric techniques appears in the following section, basic principles of visual field testing warrant mention as part of the clinical examination. Standard automated perimetry, typically using a white stimulus on a white background (white-on-white perimetry), represents the most common approach to functional assessment in glaucoma. The 24–2 or 30–2 testing patterns with the Swedish interactive threshold algorithm (SITA) provide an appropriate balance of testing efficiency and diagnostic information for most patients.

Characteristic glaucomatous field defects include paracentral scotomas, nasal steps, and arcuate defects that respect the horizontal meridian, corresponding to the pattern of damage to the optic nerve head. As disease advances, these isolated defects may coalesce into larger arcuate scotomas and eventually central island loss in end-stage disease.

Interpretation of visual field results requires consideration of reliability indices, including fixation losses, false positives, and false negatives. Global indices such as mean deviation (MD) and pattern standard deviation (PSD) provide summary measures of field loss, while the glaucoma hemifield test (GHT) specifically evaluates asymmetry across the horizontal meridian characteristic of glaucomatous damage.

Integrating Clinical Findings

The diagnosis of glaucoma rarely rests on a single examination finding but rather emerges from the integration of structural and functional assessments considered within the context of patient-specific risk factors. Characteristic structural changes at the optic nerve head with corresponding visual field defects provide the most definitive evidence of glaucomatous optic neuropathy. However, practitioners must recognize that structural and functional progression may occur asynchronously, with structural changes typically preceding detectable functional deficits in early disease.

The comprehensive clinical examination establishes the foundation for diagnosis and classification, guides appropriate further testing, and provides the baseline for monitoring progression. While advanced imaging modalities provide valuable quantitative information, they complement rather than replace the careful clinical assessment performed by an experienced examiner. The integration of these traditional clinical techniques with newer diagnostic technologies, as discussed in subsequent sections, optimizes our ability to detect glaucoma at its earliest stages and monitor progression with increasing precision.

SECTION 2—IMAGING AND TECHNOLOGICAL ADVANCES IN DIAGNOSIS

The past three decades has witnessed remarkable technological advances in glaucoma diagnostics, transforming our ability to detect early disease and monitor progression with unprecedented precision. These innovations have shifted the diagnostic paradigm from subjective assessment toward quantitative analysis of structural and functional parameters. Advanced imaging technologies provide objective, reproducible measurements of optic nerve head topography, retinal nerve fiber layer thickness, and macular ganglion cell complex integrity, often revealing damage before detectable visual field loss occurs. This section examines current imaging and technological modalities that complement traditional clinical examination in glaucoma diagnosis and management.

Optical Coherence Tomography

Optical coherence tomography (OCT) has revolutionized glaucoma imaging since its introduction in the 1990s, evolving from time-domain to spectral-domain and now swept-source technology with dramatically improved resolution and acquisition speed. OCT utilizes low-coherence interferometry to generate cross-sectional images of ocular tissues with near-histological resolution, providing detailed structural analysis of the optic nerve head, peripapillary retinal nerve fiber layer (RNFL), and macular ganglion cell complex.

Peripapillary RNFL analysis represents the most established OCT application in glaucoma, typically measured in a 3.4 mm diameter circle centered on the optic disc. RNFL thickness measurements are presented as global averages and sectoral values, commonly divided into quadrants or clock-hour segments. These measurements are compared against age-matched normative databases, with values categorized as within normal limits, borderline, or outside normal limits. The characteristic double-hump pattern of RNFL thickness (thicker superiorly and inferiorly than nasally and temporally) parallels the normal neuroretinal rim configuration, with thinning in glaucoma typically beginning in the inferotemporal and superotemporal regions.

Optic nerve head analysis provides quantitative assessment of parameters previously evaluated subjectively, including disc and cup areas, rim area, and cup-to-disc ratios. Advanced algorithms such as the Bruch's membrane opening-minimum rim width (BMO-MRW) measurement offer anatomically more precise quantification of neuroretinal rim tissue. This approach identifies the true anatomic disc margin at Bruch's membrane opening and measures the minimum distance from this boundary to the internal limiting membrane, providing a more accurate assessment of rim tissue than conventional clinical techniques.

Macular ganglion cell analysis has emerged as an important complement to peripapillary RNFL measurement, recognizing that approximately 50% of retinal ganglion cells reside in the macula. OCT segmentation algorithms can isolate and measure the ganglion cell layer (GCL) alone or in combination with the inner plexiform layer (IPL) as the ganglion cell complex. Because the macula contains minimal large retinal vessels and demonstrates less anatomic variability than the optic nerve head, macular thickness measurements may offer advantages in certain patient populations, particularly those with high myopia or tilted discs where peripapillary measurements present interpretive challenges.

Several factors influence OCT measurement reliability and interpretability. Signal strength, affected by media opacity, pupil size, and alignment, significantly impacts image quality and measurement reproducibility. Anatomic variations including high myopia, peripapillary atrophy, and small or tilted discs can confound interpretation by altering the normal distribution of retinal layers. Age-related thinning of the RNFL (approximately 0.2–0.3 µm per year) must be considered when evaluating

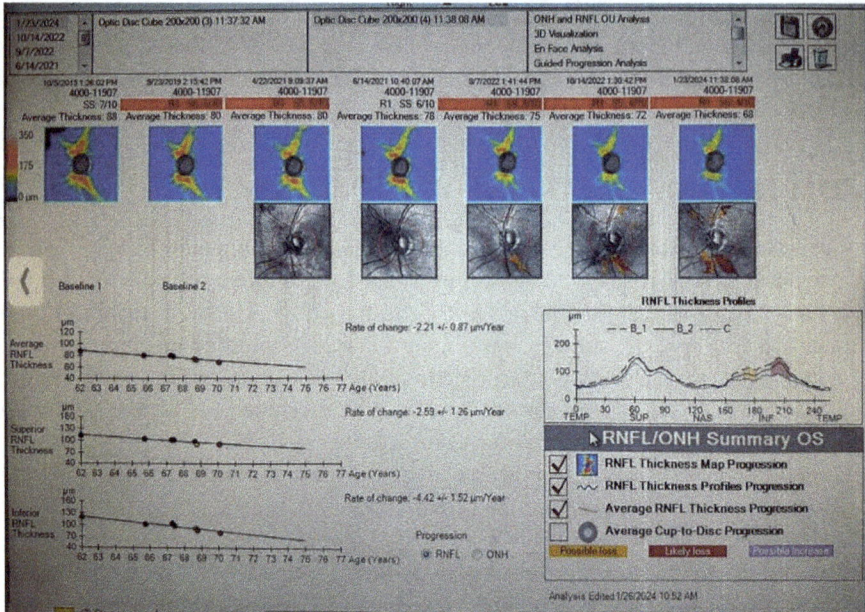

Figure 4.2 Guided progression analysis using OCT.

potential progression. Most importantly, measurements must be interpreted in clinical context, recognizing that numerous conditions beyond glaucoma can affect RNFL thickness, including demyelinating disease, ischemic optic neuropathy, and retinal vascular disorders.

Figure 4.2 demonstrates a guided progression analysis based on serial optical coherence tomography (OCT) measurements of the retinal nerve fiber layer (RNFL) in a glaucoma patient. The image highlights progressive RNFL thinning over time, underlining the essential role of OCT in monitoring structural glaucomatous damage.

OCT angiography (OCTA) represents a recent innovation that allows noninvasive visualization of the retinal and optic nerve head microvasculature without contrast injection. OCTA generates three-dimensional vascular maps by detecting temporal changes in OCT signal caused by moving blood cells. Studies have demonstrated reduced vessel density in the peripapillary and macular regions in glaucoma patients, even in early disease. Vascular parameters often correlate with structural and functional measures, suggesting potential value as complementary biomarkers for early detection and monitoring. However, the technology requires further validation before widespread clinical adoption for glaucoma management.

Confocal Scanning Laser Ophthalmoscopy

Confocal scanning laser ophthalmoscopy (CSLO), commercially available as the Heidelberg retina tomograph (HRT), constructs three-dimensional topographic images of the optic nerve head through optical sectioning. The technology captures a series of confocal images at different depths, creating a topographic map of the optic nerve surface with precise measurements of disc area, cup area, rim area, cup volume, rim volume, cup-to-disc ratio, and cup shape.

The diagnostic capability of CSLO relies on sophisticated analysis algorithms that compare patient measurements against normative databases. The Moorfields regression analysis classifies the neuroretinal rim area in six sectors as within normal limits, borderline, or outside normal limits based on the relationship between rim area and disc size in healthy subjects. The glaucoma probability score uses a machine learning classifier to calculate the probability of glaucoma based on optic nerve head morphology, independent of the contour line placement required for standard analysis.

Longitudinal analysis with CSLO provides topographic change analysis (TCA), which identifies clusters of pixels with significant height changes over time. This approach can detect subtle progressive changes in optic nerve head topography before conventional clinical assessment reveals detectable progression. However, the technology has been gradually supplanted by OCT in many clinical settings due to OCT's additional capability for retinal layer segmentation and broader applications beyond glaucoma assessment.

Scanning Laser Polarimetry

Scanning laser polarimetry (SLP), commercially implemented as the GDx, measures RNFL thickness by analyzing changes in polarization (retardation) of a laser beam as it passes through the birefringent microtubules in retinal ganglion cell axons. The retardation correlates with RNFL thickness, allowing quantitative assessment of peripapillary nerve fiber integrity.

Modern SLP incorporates enhanced corneal compensation to address the confounding effects of corneal birefringence, significantly improving diagnostic accuracy. The technology provides global and sectoral RNFL measurements along with parameters such as the nerve fiber indicator (NFI), which combines multiple measurements into a single value indicating the likelihood of glaucomatous damage. While studies have demonstrated comparable diagnostic performance between SLP and other imaging modalities, this technology has become less commonly utilized in clinical practice with the widespread adoption of OCT.

Fundus Photography and Computer-Aided Image Analysis

Digital fundus photography provides permanent documentation of optic nerve head appearance, enabling side-by-side comparison over time to detect subtle changes in neuroretinal rim configuration, disc hemorrhages, or peripapillary atrophy. Stereoscopic photography offers enhanced appreciation of the three-dimensional structure of the optic nerve head, although expertise in stereoscopic interpretation is increasingly uncommon.

Computer-aided image analysis of fundus photographs has evolved to include automated detection of the optic disc margin, cup boundary, and cup-to-disc ratio estimation. Modern systems incorporate deep learning algorithms to identify features associated with glaucomatous damage, potentially enhancing detection sensitivity and reducing inter-observer variability. Advances in ultra-widefield imaging also facilitate documentation of peripheral retinal pathology that may contribute to secondary glaucoma.

Anterior Segment Imaging

Technological advances in anterior segment imaging have significantly enhanced evaluation of the angle structures critical for accurate glaucoma classification and management. Anterior segment optical coherence tomography (AS-OCT) provides cross-sectional images of the anterior chamber, allowing quantitative assessment of angle configuration, iris profile, and anterior chamber dimensions. This technology offers advantages over gonioscopy, including non-contact imaging, objective measurements, and visualization through opaque corneas.

AS-OCT enables quantification of parameters such as angle opening distance, trabecular-iris space area, and angle recess area, which correlate with risk for angle closure. The technology facilitates identification of mechanisms contributing to angle closure, including pupillary block, plateau iris configuration, and lens-induced component, guiding appropriate intervention selection. While AS-OCT provides valuable objective documentation, it currently complements rather than replaces gonioscopy, which offers dynamic assessment and better visualization of angle structures such as peripheral anterior synechiae.

Ultrasound biomicroscopy (UBM) utilizes high-frequency ultrasound to generate high-resolution images of anterior segment structures, including regions behind the iris plane inaccessible to OCT due to limited penetration through pigmented tissues. UBM excels in visualizing the ciliary body, lens zonules, and posterior chamber, making it particularly valuable for evaluating plateau iris syndrome, ciliary body effusion, and lens-related angle closure mechanisms. The technology requires immersion technique with a water bath or coupling gel, limiting its routine application compared to non-contact methods.

Figure 4.3 illustrates a plateau iris configuration captured by ultrasound biomicroscopy (UBM). This anatomical variant is characterized by anteriorly positioned ciliary processes that narrow the anterior chamber angle despite a deep central chamber, contributing to angle-closure pathogenesis.

Advanced Perimetry

While standard automated perimetry (SAP) remains the clinical standard for functional assessment in glaucoma, novel perimetric technologies aim to detect functional deficits earlier in the disease process by targeting specific ganglion cell subpopulations or using alternative testing strategies. Frequency doubling technology (FDT) perimetry presents low spatial frequency sinusoidal gratings undergoing rapid phase reversal, creating an illusion of doubled spatial frequency. This stimulus preferentially stimulates the magnocellular pathway and non-linear retinal ganglion cells, potentially revealing damage before standard perimetry. The test demonstrates high sensitivity for moderate to advanced glaucoma, with

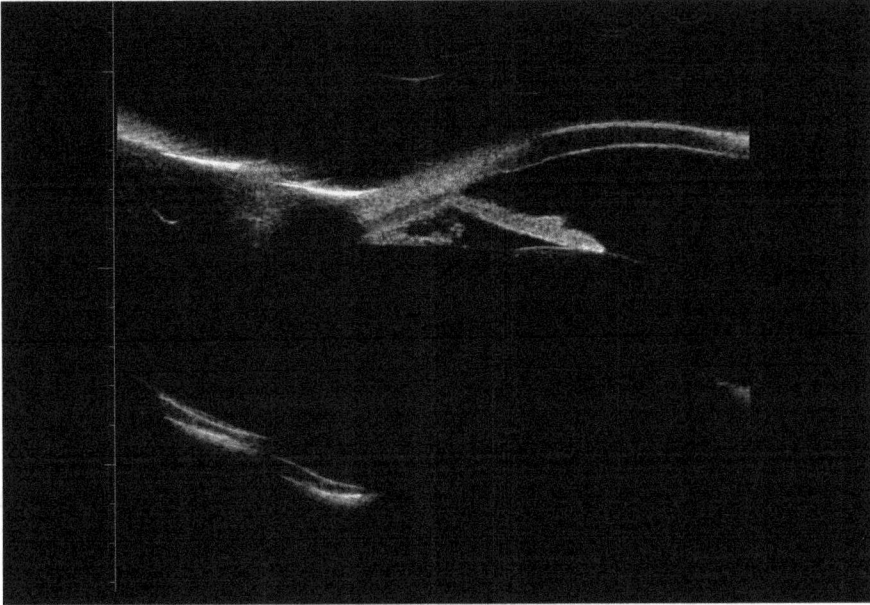

Figure 4.3 Plateau iris configuration in ultrasound biomicroscopy.

advantages including resistance to blur and cataract effects, rapid testing time, and minimal learning curve. Short-wavelength automated perimetry (SWAP) isolates and tests the blue-yellow pathway by presenting a blue stimulus on a bright yellow background, theoretically detecting damage to this vulnerable pathway earlier than conventional perimetry. However, the test's clinical adoption has been limited by increased testing time, greater variability, and significant influence of media opacity.

Flicker perimetry, which tests temporal processing by presenting a flickering stimulus, and motion perimetry, which evaluates motion detection thresholds, represent additional specialized techniques targeting functional pathways potentially affected early in glaucoma. These technologies remain primarily research tools, with insufficient evidence to support routine clinical implementation.

Artificial Intelligence in Glaucoma Diagnosis

Artificial intelligence, particularly deep learning approaches, has emerged as a powerful tool for analyzing the complex multimodal data generated in glaucoma assessment. Convolutional neural networks trained on thousands of labeled images can automatically detect features associated with glaucomatous damage in fundus photographs, OCT scans, and visual fields, often achieving diagnostic performance comparable to expert clinicians.

AI-based systems offer potential advantages including automated screening of at-risk populations, reduction in interpretation variability, integration of structural and functional data for comprehensive assessment, and identification of subtle patterns unrecognizable to human observers. Early studies suggest these systems

Table 4.1 Diagnostic Tools Used in Glaucoma Assessment

Test/Tool	What It Measures	Strength	Limitation
Tonometry	Intraocular pressure	Widely available	Diurnal variation affects results
Gonioscopy	Angle status	Gold standard for angle assessment	Operator-dependent
Perimetry	Visual field defects	Functional damage detection	Subjective, requires patient cooperation
OCT	Retinal nerve fiber layer (RNFL) thickness	Early structural damage detection	Artifacts in high myopia
Optic Disc Photography	Optic nerve head appearance	Longitudinal documentation	Less sensitive to early damage

may identify glaucomatous damage with high sensitivity and specificity, potentially facilitating earlier detection and intervention. However, challenges including dataset bias, generalizability across diverse populations, and integration into clinical workflows must be addressed before widespread implementation. Additionally, these systems currently function as decision support tools rather than replacements for clinical judgment, emphasizing the continued importance of experienced clinician oversight in glaucoma diagnosis and management.

Table 4.1 provides a comparative summary of the principal diagnostic techniques used in glaucoma assessment. It outlines what each test measures, along with their specific strengths and limitations, helping guide the choice of appropriate diagnostic strategies in various clinical scenarios.

SECTION 3—DIFFERENTIATING GLAUCOMA FROM OTHER CONDITIONS

The accurate diagnosis of glaucoma requires careful differentiation from numerous conditions that can mimic its structural and functional characteristics. Misdiagnosis may lead to unnecessary treatment with potential side effects, financial burden, and psychological impact, or conversely, missed opportunities for early intervention in true glaucomatous disease. This diagnostic challenge is compounded by the considerable overlap in clinical presentation between glaucoma and various optic neuropathies, congenital anomalies, and artifacts in structural and functional testing. This section explores the key differential diagnoses for glaucoma and provides clinical strategies for distinguishing these entities.

Physiological Optic Disc Variations

Physiological variations in optic nerve head appearance represent a common source of diagnostic uncertainty. Large physiological cups, particularly in myopic eyes or those with large optic discs, may be misinterpreted as glaucomatous. While glaucomatous damage typically manifests as vertical enlargement of the cup with preferential thinning of the superior and inferior neuroretinal rim, physiological cupping generally exhibits a more uniform, circular configuration with preservation of the normal rim contour. Furthermore, physiological cupping remains stable over time, lacking the progressive changes characteristic of glaucoma.

Tilted disc syndrome, more prevalent in myopic individuals, presents with an oblique insertion of the optic nerve, inferior ectasia, and superotemporal visual field defects that may cross the horizontal midline, distinguishing them from the typical glaucomatous pattern that respects the horizontal meridian. The presence of situs inversus of the retinal vessels and relative preservation of the neuroretinal rim further differentiate this entity from glaucoma.

Optic nerve head drusen, calcific deposits within the optic nerve substance, may produce pseudo-papilledema with elevated, lumpy disc margins, anomalous vascular branching, and absent spontaneous venous pulsation. Unlike glaucoma, drusen typically manifest with preserved central rim tissue and nasal visual field defects that tend to be stable or slowly progressive. B-scan ultrasonography, autofluorescence imaging, and enhanced-depth OCT facilitate identification of drusen, particularly when buried beneath the disc surface.

Morning glory disc anomaly, colobomatous defects, and other congenital disc variations can present with excavated optic nerves resembling glaucomatous cupping. The presence of associated features such as peripapillary pigmentary changes, vascular anomalies, and systemic associations helps distinguish these conditions. Importantly, these congenital variations typically remain stable over time, lacking the progressive nature of glaucomatous optic neuropathy.

Non-Glaucomatous Optic Neuropathies

Anterior ischemic optic neuropathy (AION), both arteritic and non-arteritic forms, may result in optic disc cupping that can mimic glaucomatous damage. Key differentiating features include the history of acute vision loss, altitudinal rather than arcuate visual field defects, pallor disproportionate to cupping, and lack of progressive change after the initial event. In arteritic AION, associated systemic symptoms, elevated inflammatory markers, and chalky-white disc appearance further distinguish this entity from glaucoma.

Compressive optic neuropathy from orbital or intracranial tumors can produce disc cupping resembling glaucoma, often with greater pallor than expected for the degree of excavation. Visual field testing may reveal defects that respect the vertical rather than horizontal meridian, and central vision is often affected earlier than in glaucoma. Neuroimaging is indicated when asymmetric or atypical disc appearance and visual field defects raise suspicion for a compressive lesion.

Hereditary optic neuropathies, including dominant optic atrophy and Leber's hereditary optic neuropathy, can present with disc cupping and excavation. Dominant optic atrophy typically manifests with bilateral temporal pallor, central or cecocentral scotomas, and a strong family history. Leber's hereditary optic neuropathy classically affects young adult males with sequential, painless central vision loss, initially presenting with peripapillary telangiectasia followed by optic atrophy. Genetic testing can confirm these diagnoses in appropriate clinical settings.

Traumatic optic neuropathy may result in optic atrophy with excavation resembling glaucomatous cupping. The history of trauma, associated orbital findings, and temporal relationship between the injury and vision loss help differentiate this entity from glaucoma. Similarly, toxic and nutritional optic neuropathies from substances such as ethambutol, methanol, or nutritional deficiencies typically present with symmetric central or cecocentral visual field defects and temporal disc pallor, distinguishing them from the peripheral field loss and superior/inferior rim thinning characteristic of glaucoma.

Neurological Conditions Affecting Visual Fields

Numerous neurological conditions can produce visual field defects that may be misinterpreted as glaucomatous. Lesions of the post-chiasmal visual pathway, including occipital lobe infarctions, tumors, or demyelinating disease, typically produce homonymous hemianopic defects that respect the vertical meridian, contrasting with the arcuate or nasal step defects in glaucoma that respect the horizontal meridian. However, chiasmal lesions such as pituitary adenomas may produce bitemporal hemianopic defects that can sometimes be confused with advanced glaucomatous field loss, particularly when asymmetric.

Migraine-associated visual field defects, often transient and migratory, can occasionally manifest as stable, non-progressive scotomas that may be mistaken for glaucomatous damage. The temporal association with headache, younger age of onset, and lack of corresponding optic nerve changes help distinguish these functional defects from true glaucomatous loss.

Functional (non-organic) visual field loss presents with characteristic patterns including tunnel vision (constriction unaffected by test distance), crossing of isopters, or spiraling on manual perimetry. Automated perimetry may reveal high false positive responses, inconsistent responses to stimuli of different intensities, or excessively high threshold values in severely constricted fields. The absence of corresponding structural damage and lack of progression over time are key to identifying non-organic visual loss.

Pigmentary Retinopathies and Chorioretinal Disorders

Retinitis pigmentosa and related pigmentary retinopathies can produce visual field constriction that may be confused with advanced glaucoma, particularly when disc pallor is present. The characteristic bone-spicule pigmentation, attenuated vessels, electroretinographic abnormalities, and family history facilitate differentiation. Similarly, chorioretinal disorders such as white dot syndromes or posterior uveitis may result in visual field defects that could be misattributed to glaucoma in the absence of careful fundus examination.

Age-related macular degeneration (AMD) can produce central or paracentral scotomas that occasionally mimic glaucomatous field loss, particularly when testing reliability is limited. The presence of drusen, pigmentary changes, or choroidal neovascularization on fundus examination, along with preserved neuroretinal rim, distinguishes AMD from glaucoma.

Imaging Artifacts and Limitations

Modern imaging modalities, while providing valuable diagnostic information, can introduce artifacts that may lead to misinterpretation. OCT artifacts commonly result from segmentation errors, particularly in eyes with high myopia, peripapillary atrophy, or vitreoretinal interface abnormalities. Signal strength reduction from media opacity or misalignment can produce falsely thinned measurements suggesting glaucomatous damage. Careful review of the scan quality, segmentation accuracy, and correlation with clinical findings is essential to avoid misdiagnosis based on imaging artifacts.

Normative database limitations affect all imaging modalities, with reduced accuracy for patients at the extremes of refractive error, age, or optic disc size. Many databases underrepresent certain ethnic groups, potentially reducing diagnostic precision in these populations. Recognition of these limitations is crucial for appropriate interpretation of quantitative imaging results in the context of the clinical examination.

Integrated Diagnostic Approach

Differentiating glaucoma from its mimics requires an integrated approach combining detailed clinical examination with appropriate ancillary testing. Several principles guide this diagnostic strategy.

Structure-function correlation represents a fundamental concept in glaucoma diagnosis. True glaucomatous damage typically demonstrates congruence between the location of structural abnormalities (e.g., focal neuroretinal rim thinning or RNFL defects) and functional deficits on visual field testing. Discordance between structural and functional findings should prompt consideration of non-glaucomatous etiologies.

Longitudinal evaluation documenting progression remains the gold standard for confirming glaucomatous disease. While many conditions can resemble glaucoma on initial presentation, the progressive nature of untreated glaucoma distinguishes it from most static optic neuropathies or congenital variations. Careful documentation of optic nerve appearance, imaging measurements, and visual field parameters over time facilitates detection of subtle progressive changes indicative of glaucoma.

Comprehensive assessment requires consideration of the entire clinical picture rather than isolated test results. Patient age, risk factors, family history, systemic health, and medication use provide important context for interpreting examination findings. Atypical features such as disproportionate visual acuity loss, color vision deficits, pain, or neurologic symptoms should trigger investigation for alternative diagnoses.

By applying these principles and maintaining awareness of the various conditions that can mimic glaucoma, clinicians can optimize diagnostic accuracy, avoiding both unnecessary treatment and missed opportunities for appropriate intervention in this potentially blinding disease.

CHAPTER 5
MEDICAL MANAGEMENT OF GLAUCOMA

Despite remarkable advances in surgical techniques and laser technology, pharmacological therapy remains the cornerstone of glaucoma management for most patients worldwide. Medical therapy offers a noninvasive approach to intraocular pressure reduction, the only proven modifiable risk factor for slowing glaucomatous progression. The landscape of glaucoma pharmacotherapy has evolved significantly over the past several decades, from relatively limited options with substantial side effect profiles to an expanded armamentarium of more targeted, potent, and better-tolerated medications. This evolution has enabled more personalized treatment approaches that consider not only efficacy but also safety, convenience, cost, and individual patient characteristics.

The primary objective of glaucoma medical management is to achieve a target intraocular pressure at which disease progression is halted or sufficiently slowed to maintain visual function and quality of life throughout the patient's lifetime. This goal-oriented approach requires careful consideration of disease severity, rate of progression, risk factors, life expectancy, and individual patient circumstances. Pharmacological agents with diverse mechanisms of action offer various approaches to modulating aqueous humor dynamics, either by reducing production or enhancing outflow through conventional and unconventional pathways.

While the efficacy of medications in lowering intraocular pressure is well-established, the clinical effectiveness of treatment depends significantly on patient adherence and persistence with therapy. The chronic, often asymptomatic nature of glaucoma presents unique challenges to medication compliance, necessitating strategies to address barriers at the patient, provider, and healthcare system levels. The disconnect between controlled clinical trial efficacy and real-world effectiveness highlights the importance of practical approaches to optimizing medical therapy.

This chapter explores different aspects of glaucoma pharmacotherapy, beginning with an overview of medication classes and their roles in contemporary management paradigms. It then examines the specific mechanisms of action of anti-glaucoma medications and their implications for therapeutic selection and combination strategies. The final section addresses the critical challenge of patient compliance, exploring factors affecting adherence and evidence-based approaches to enhancing medication-taking behavior. By integrating pharmacological knowledge with practical clinical considerations, this chapter aims to provide a comprehensive framework for optimizing medical management in patients with glaucoma.

DOI: 10.1201/9781003646693-5

SECTION 1—OVERVIEW OF PHARMACOLOGICAL THERAPIES

Medical therapy for glaucoma has undergone remarkable evolution since the introduction of pilocarpine in the late 19th century. Today's clinicians benefit from a diverse array of pharmacological agents that target different aspects of aqueous humor dynamics to achieve intraocular pressure (IOP) reduction. This section provides a comprehensive overview of the major drug classes used in glaucoma management, their clinical applications, comparative efficacy, and considerations for initial therapy selection and stepwise treatment escalation.

Major Classes of Glaucoma Medications

The pharmacological options for glaucoma management can be categorized into five major classes based on their mechanisms and chemical structures: prostaglandin analogs, beta-adrenergic antagonists, alpha-adrenergic agonists, carbonic anhydrase inhibitors, and cholinergic agents. Additionally, fixed-dose combination medications that incorporate two or more active ingredients in a single formulation represent an increasingly important component of the therapeutic armamentarium.

Prostaglandin analogs (PGAs) have emerged as first-line therapy for most forms of open-angle glaucoma and ocular hypertension. This class includes latanoprost, travoprost, bimatoprost, and tafluprost. PGAs typically reduce IOP by 25–35% from baseline, with once-daily dosing that enhances convenience and compliance. Their favorable systemic safety profile, with minimal effects on cardiovascular and pulmonary function, contributes to their preferential status in initial therapy. However, ocular side effects including conjunctival hyperemia, periorbital fat atrophy, iris darkening, and eyelash growth must be discussed with patients. Recent additions to this class include latanoprostene bunod, which incorporates a nitric oxide-donating moiety to enhance conventional outflow facility beyond that achieved with traditional PGAs.

Beta-adrenergic antagonists (beta-blockers) were the mainstay of glaucoma therapy prior to the introduction of PGAs and remain important second-line or adjunctive agents. This class includes non-selective agents (timolol, levobunolol, carteolol) and cardioselective options (betaxolol). Beta-blockers typically reduce IOP by 20–25% from baseline, with twice-daily dosing for most formulations, though some gel-forming solutions allow once-daily administration. Their systemic side effect profile—including bradycardia, bronchospasm, depression, and masking of hypoglycemic symptoms—necessitates careful patient selection and monitoring. According to a comprehensive review despite being supplanted as first-line therapy, beta-blockers remain among the most frequently prescribed glaucoma medications worldwide due to their effectiveness and relatively low cost (29).

Alpha-adrenergic agonists include brimonidine and apraclonidine, with the former more commonly used for chronic therapy due to lower rates of tachyphylaxis and allergic reactions. These agents typically reduce IOP by 15–25% from baseline and require dosing two to three times daily. Brimonidine's potential neuroprotective properties, suggested in animal models, have generated interest beyond its IOP-lowering effects, though clinical evidence for neuroprotection in humans remains inconclusive. Ocular side effects include hyperemia, allergic conjunctivitis (in up to 30% of patients with long-term use), and follicular conjunctivitis. Systemic effects such as fatigue, dry mouth, and hypotension occur less frequently than with older, less selective alpha-agonists but remain considerations in elderly patients.

Carbonic anhydrase inhibitors (CAIs) are available in both topical (dorzolamide, brinzolamide) and oral (acetazolamide, methazolamide) formulations. Topical CAIs typically reduce IOP by 15–20% from baseline and require dosing two to three times daily. These agents are particularly valuable as adjunctive therapy and in patients with contraindications to other medication classes. Ocular side effects include stinging, burning, and bitter taste after installation. Oral CAIs produce greater IOP reduction (20–30%) but with more significant systemic side effects, including paresthesias, fatigue, gastrointestinal disturbances, metabolic acidosis, and rarely, blood dyscrasias or nephrolithiasis. Consequently, oral formulations are typically reserved for short-term use in acute pressure elevation or as temporizing measures before surgical intervention in refractory cases.

Cholinergic agents (miotics), primarily pilocarpine, were among the earliest medications used for glaucoma but have been largely supplanted by newer agents with more favorable dosing regimens and side effect profiles. These agents reduce IOP by 15–25% from baseline and require dosing three to four times daily. Visual side effects, including induced myopia, decreased vision in dim illumination, and brow ache, significantly limit patient acceptance, particularly in younger individuals with preserved accommodation. Nonetheless, these medications retain a role in specific scenarios such as acute angle-closure, plateau iris syndrome, and some cases of pigmentary glaucoma.

Fixed-dose combination medications have gained prominence in contemporary glaucoma management, addressing challenges of polypharmacy, preservative exposure, compliance, and washout effects from multiple medications. Current combinations predominantly pair a beta-blocker (typically timolol) with a second agent from another class (PGA, CAI, or alpha-agonist). More recently, preservative-free formulations and combinations without beta-blockers have expanded options for patients with specific contraindications or intolerances. A network meta-analysis (30) demonstrated that fixed combinations typically offer slightly reduced efficacy compared to unfixed concomitant therapy with the same components, though this difference is often outweighed by improved convenience and adherence.

Comparative Efficacy and Approach to Initial Therapy

The selection of initial therapy requires consideration of multiple factors including efficacy, safety profile, dosing convenience, cost, and patient-specific characteristics. Evidence consistently demonstrates that PGAs offer superior IOP reduction as monotherapy compared to other classes, with the additional advantages of once-daily dosing and minimal systemic side effects. These factors underlie their position as preferred first-line agents in major treatment guidelines.

However, individualized therapy remains paramount, as certain clinical scenarios may favor alternative initial approaches. For example, beta-blockers may be preferred in unilateral disease where the cosmetic effects of PGAs are concerning, in young patients with milder IOP elevation, or in regions where cost constraints limit access to newer agents. Alpha-agonists or CAIs may be selected for initial therapy in patients with contraindications to both PGAs and beta-blockers, though their less robust efficacy and more frequent dosing must be considered.

Stepwise Therapy and Maximizing Medical Treatment

When initial monotherapy fails to achieve target IOP or disease progression continues despite pressure reduction, stepwise escalation of therapy follows several general principles:

- *First*, ensuring adequate trial duration and monitoring adherence with initial therapy before concluding treatment failure is essential. For most agents, peak efficacy occurs within 3–4 weeks of initiation, though PGAs may require up to 6–8 weeks for maximal effect.
- *Second*, when considering additional therapy, selecting agents with complementary mechanisms of action typically provides more additive pressure reduction than combining drugs that work through similar pathways. For example, adding a CAI or alpha-agonist to a PGA generally offers greater additional reduction than combining a PGA with another outflow-enhancing medication.
- *Third*, with each medication added, the incremental benefit typically diminishes while the burden of side effects, cost, and complexity increases. The first adjunctive medication may provide an additional 15–20% reduction from the new baseline, while subsequent additions often yield progressively smaller benefits.
- *Fourth*, fixed-combination formulations should be considered when patients require multiple medications, particularly when adherence concerns exist or ocular surface disease from preservative exposure becomes problematic.
- *Finally*, the concept of maximum medical therapy has evolved from the historical "shotgun" approach of prescribing one medication from each class toward more nuanced, individualized assessment of risk–benefit ratios. Contemporary maximum medical therapy typically involves two to three medications (often including a fixed combination) selected based on efficacy, tolerability, and adherence considerations, rather than indiscriminate use of all available classes.

Special Populations and Considerations

Certain patient populations require modified approaches to pharmacological management. In pregnant women, the risk–benefit assessment changes substantially, with most glaucoma medications carrying pregnancy category C or B designations. When treatment is necessary, beta-blockers (particularly timolol gel) or brimonidine are often selected, with careful consideration of timing and technique to minimize systemic absorption.

In pediatric glaucoma patients, medical therapy frequently serves as an adjunct to surgical intervention rather than primary treatment. When medications are needed, beta-blockers and CAIs are commonly employed, while PGAs demonstrate variable and often reduced efficacy in congenital and juvenile glaucoma compared to adult forms.

Elderly patients with multiple comorbidities require careful consideration of potential drug interactions and systemic side effects. In this population, PGAs often remain preferred initial therapy due to minimal systemic effects, though ensuring proper instillation technique may present challenges with arthritis or limited dexterity.

In normal-tension glaucoma, medical therapy remains a cornerstone of management despite the normal baseline pressures. Studies suggest that IOP reduction of 30% from baseline significantly reduces progression risk, with similar medication efficacy patterns to high-pressure glaucoma, though achieving this target often requires multiple medications.

The expanded pharmacological armamentarium for glaucoma has enabled more personalized, effective management strategies while presenting challenges in selecting optimal regimens from numerous available options. Understanding the relative efficacy, safety profiles, and practical considerations of each medication class provides the foundation for evidence-based, patient-centered treatment decisions. As newer agents and innovative delivery systems continue to emerge, the principles of individualized therapy selection, stepwise treatment escalation, and careful monitoring of both efficacy and tolerability remain fundamental to optimizing outcomes in medical management of glaucoma.

SECTION 2—MECHANISMS OF ACTION OF ANTI-GLAUCOMA DRUGS

Understanding the mechanisms by which anti-glaucoma medications lower intraocular pressure (IOP) provides the pharmacological foundation for rational therapeutic selection and combination strategies. These mechanisms broadly involve modulation of aqueous humor dynamics through two principal pathways: decreasing aqueous production or enhancing aqueous outflow. This section examines the specific molecular and cellular mechanisms underlying the action of each major drug class, their effects on ocular physiology, and the pharmacological basis for their clinical efficacy and side effect profiles.

Aqueous humor, produced by the ciliary epithelium at a rate of approximately 2–3 $\mu L/min$, maintains proper IOP, provides nutritional support to avascular ocular structures, and removes metabolic waste products. The balance between aqueous production and outflow determines IOP, creating a critical target for pharmacological intervention. Understanding normal aqueous physiology provides essential context for drug mechanisms. Aqueous production involves three primary processes: active secretion (responsible for 80–90% of formation), ultrafiltration, and diffusion. Active secretion depends on energy-dependent ion transporters, primarily Na^+-K^+-ATPase and carbonic anhydrase enzymes, which create osmotic gradients driving aqueous movement. Aqueous outflow occurs through two pathways: the conventional (trabecular) pathway, which is pressure-dependent and accounts for approximately 80–90% of outflow in healthy eyes, and the unconventional (uveoscleral) pathway, which is relatively pressure-independent and responsible for the remaining 10–20% of outflow. Glaucoma medications target various aspects of these physiological processes to modulate aqueous dynamics and reduce IOP.

Prostaglandin Analogs: Enhancing Uveoscleral Outflow

Prostaglandin analogs (PGAs) primarily reduce IOP by increasing aqueous outflow through the unconventional uveoscleral pathway, with emerging evidence suggesting additional effects on conventional outflow facility. These lipid-derived compounds act as prodrugs, requiring enzymatic hydrolysis by corneal esterases to their active free acid forms. Upon reaching their target tissues in the anterior segment, PGAs bind to specific prostanoid receptors, predominantly the FP receptor (prostaglandin F receptor), initiating a cascade of cellular events. The primary mechanism involves remodeling of the extracellular matrix in the ciliary muscle and uveoscleral tissues. PGAs induce upregulation of matrix metalloproteinases (MMPs), particularly MMP-1, MMP-2, MMP-3, and MMP-9, as demonstrated in both laboratory studies and clinical samples from PGA-treated patients. These enzymes degrade collagen types I, III, and IV within the extracellular matrix of the ciliary muscle and sclera, reducing hydraulic resistance to aqueous flow through these tissues. Additionally, PGAs reduce collagen synthesis in the ciliary muscle, further contributing to the altered extracellular environment that facilitates increased uveoscleral outflow.

Recent studies suggest that PGAs also enhance conventional outflow through effects on the trabecular meshwork and Schlemm's canal. Existing research (31) has demonstrated that PGAs increase permeability of Schlemm's canal endothelial cells through reorganization of the cellular cytoskeleton and junctional proteins, potentially increasing conventional outflow facility. This dual mechanism may explain the robust and sustained IOP-lowering efficacy of this drug class.

The molecular basis for PGA-associated side effects reflects their effects on various tissues. Conjunctival hyperemia results from nitric oxide-mediated vasodilation triggered by prostaglandin receptor activation in conjunctival vessels. Iris darkening occurs through increased melanin synthesis in iris melanocytes, induced by FP receptor stimulation and subsequent upregulation of tyrosinase, the rate-limiting enzyme in melanogenesis. Periorbital fat atrophy and enophthalmos likely result from FP receptor-mediated inhibition of adipocyte differentiation and proliferation, along with MMP-mediated degradation of orbital connective tissues. Eyelash growth (trichomegaly) reflects PGA-induced stimulation of follicular cells, shifting hair follicles into the growth phase of their cycle.

Newer additions to the PGA class, such as latanoprostene bunod, incorporate nitric oxide-donating moieties that enhance conventional outflow through trabecular meshwork and Schlemm's canal cells. Nitric oxide activates guanylate cyclase, increasing intracellular cGMP, which leads to relaxation of trabecular meshwork cells and increased permeability of Schlemm's canal, providing additive IOP reduction beyond traditional PGAs.

Beta-Adrenergic Antagonists: Reducing Aqueous Production

Beta-adrenergic antagonists (beta-blockers) lower IOP primarily by decreasing aqueous humor production, with minimal effects on outflow facility. These agents competitively block beta-adrenergic receptors on the non-pigmented ciliary epithelium, inhibiting the stimulatory effects of endogenous catecholamines (epinephrine and norepinephrine) on aqueous secretion.

At the molecular level, beta-blockers prevent catecholamine-induced activation of adenylate cyclase, thereby reducing intracellular cyclic adenosine monophosphate (cAMP) levels. Decreased cAMP leads to reduced activity of protein kinase A, which normally phosphorylates and activates key proteins involved in aqueous secretion, including Na^+-K^+-ATPase and other ion transporters. This ultimately decreases active ion transport across the ciliary epithelium, reducing the osmotic gradient that drives aqueous formation.

Non-selective beta-blockers (timolol, levobunolol, carteolol) inhibit both β_1 and β_2 receptors, while cardioselective agents (betaxolol) primarily block β_1 receptors. In ocular tissues, β_2 receptors predominate, explaining the somewhat reduced efficacy of betaxolol compared to non-selective agents. However, the higher β_1 selectivity provides a more favorable systemic safety profile in patients with respiratory conditions, as β_2 receptors mediate bronchodilation.

Interestingly, the IOP-lowering effect of beta-blockers demonstrates diurnal variation, with greater efficacy during daytime hours and reduced nighttime efficacy. This pattern reflects the circadian rhythm of endogenous catecholamine production, which peaks during waking hours. During sleep, when sympathetic tone is reduced, less endogenous receptor stimulation occurs, resulting in limited additional benefit from receptor blockade. This phenomenon, through a 24-hour IOP monitoring study (32), explains why beta-blockers may inadequately control nocturnal IOP and supports the rationale for combination therapy with agents working through different mechanisms.

The systemic side effects of beta-blockers directly relate to their receptor-blocking actions in non-ocular tissues. Bronchospasm results from β_2 receptor blockade in bronchial smooth muscle, bradycardia from β_1 receptor blockade in cardiac tissue, and hypotension from combined effects on cardiac output and peripheral vascular resistance. Central nervous system effects, including depression, fatigue, and memory impairment, likely result from beta-blocker penetration across the blood-brain barrier, particularly with more lipophilic agents.

Alpha-Adrenergic Agonists: Dual Mechanism of Action

Alpha-adrenergic agonists exhibit a dual mechanism of action, initially reducing aqueous production and subsequently enhancing uveoscleral outflow. Brimonidine, the predominant agent in this class for chronic glaucoma therapy, selectively activates α_2-adrenergic receptors, which function as presynaptic autoreceptors regulating neurotransmitter release as well as postsynaptic effector receptors in target tissues. In the ciliary epithelium, α_2-receptor activation inhibits adenylate cyclase, reducing cAMP levels and decreasing aqueous humor production through mechanisms similar to beta-blockers. This effect accounts for the immediate IOP reduction observed within 1–2 hours after instillation. With chronic administration, increased uveoscleral outflow becomes the predominant mechanism, mediated through α_2-receptor-induced upregulation of prostaglandin synthesis and subsequent extracellular matrix remodeling in the ciliary muscle, albeit less extensively than with direct PGA therapy.

The systemic effects of alpha-agonists reflect the distribution of α_2-receptors throughout the body. Fatigue and dry mouth result from central nervous system α_2-receptor activation, which reduces norepinephrine release in the locus coeruleus and salivary glands, respectively. The potential neuroprotective properties suggested for brimonidine involve multiple pathways, including inhibition of glutamate release, upregulation of brain-derived neurotrophic factor (BDNF), and activation of anti-apoptotic genes, though definitive clinical evidence for these effects remains limited.

Selective α_2-agonists represent a significant improvement over earlier non-selective agents like apraclonidine and epinephrine, which activate both α_1 and α_2 receptors. α_1-receptor activation produces vasoconstriction and mydriasis, undesirable effects for chronic glaucoma therapy. The approximately 1000-fold greater selectivity of brimonidine for α_2 versus α_1 receptors explains its superior side effect profile and reduced tachyphylaxis compared to less selective agents.

Carbonic Anhydrase Inhibitors: Disrupting Aqueous Formation

Carbonic anhydrase inhibitors (CAIs) reduce aqueous humor production by inhibiting the catalytic activity of carbonic anhydrase (CA) enzymes, particularly the CA-II and CA-IV isoforms present in the ciliary epithelium. These enzymes catalyze the reversible hydration of carbon dioxide to form carbonic acid, which dissociates into bicarbonate and hydrogen ions:

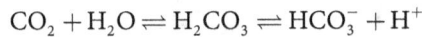

$$CO_2 + H_2O \rightleftharpoons H_2CO_3 \rightleftharpoons HCO_3^- + H^+$$

This reaction is critical for generating bicarbonate ions that, along with sodium ions, create the osmotic gradient driving aqueous humor formation. By inhibiting CA activity, these drugs reduce bicarbonate formation, decrease active sodium and fluid transport, and consequently lower the rate of aqueous production by approximately 40–60%. The sulfonamide moiety common to all CAIs binds to the zinc atom at the active site of the enzyme, preventing substrate access and catalytic activity. The different pharmacokinetic properties of topical versus systemic CAIs reflect their distribution and access to various CA isoenzymes. Topical agents (dorzolamide, brinzolamide) primarily affect the membrane-bound CA-IV isoenzyme accessible from the ocular surface, while systemic CAIs (acetazolamide, methazolamide) reach the cytosolic CA-II isoenzyme through the bloodstream, potentially offering more complete enzyme inhibition and explaining their somewhat greater efficacy.

The systemic side effects of CAIs directly relate to the inhibition of CA isoenzymes throughout the body. Metabolic acidosis results from reduced bicarbonate reabsorption in the renal tubules, while paresthesias, fatigue, and altered taste sensation reflect altered pH and electrolyte balance in neural tissues and taste buds. Topical CAIs produce minimal systemic carbonic anhydrase inhibition at therapeutic doses, explaining their improved systemic safety profile compared to oral agents.

Cholinergic Agents: Enhancing Conventional Outflow

Cholinergic agents, including direct-acting parasympathomimetics (pilocarpine, carbachol) and cholinesterase inhibitors (echothiophate, demecarium), lower IOP by increasing aqueous outflow through the conventional trabecular pathway. These drugs stimulate muscarinic acetylcholine receptors (primarily M3 subtype) on the ciliary muscle, causing contraction that physically alters the configuration of the trabecular meshwork and Schlemm's canal. Ciliary muscle contraction creates mechanical tension on the scleral spur and trabecular meshwork, expanding intertrabecular spaces and reducing resistance to aqueous flow. Additionally, contraction of the longitudinal portion of the ciliary muscle opens the trabecular lamellae and dilates Schlemm's canal, further facilitating conventional outflow. Direct measurement of outflow facility demonstrates a 2–4-fold increase with pilocarpine administration.

The side effects of cholinergic agents directly relate to muscarinic receptor stimulation in various ocular tissues. Pupillary miosis results from contraction of the iris sphincter muscle, induced ciliary muscle contraction causes accommodative spasm with resultant myopic shift, and stimulation of conjunctival goblet cells increases mucus secretion. Rarely, systemic effects including bradycardia, hypotension, and bronchospasm may occur with sufficient drug absorption, reflecting muscarinic receptor activation in cardiac, vascular, and pulmonary tissues.

Rho-Kinase Inhibitors: Novel Mechanisms for Trabecular Outflow Enhancement

The newest class of glaucoma medications, Rho-kinase (ROCK) inhibitors, represents a significant innovation in targeting the conventional outflow pathway directly. These agents inhibit Rho-associated protein kinase, a serine/threonine kinase that regulates cellular contractility, motility, and morphology through effects on the actin cytoskeleton.

In the trabecular meshwork, ROCK inhibition leads to relaxation of trabecular meshwork cells, reduced cell contractility, and altered cell-matrix adhesions, collectively increasing permeability and reducing outflow resistance. Additionally, these agents enhance Schlemm's canal endothelial cell permeability by reducing cell stiffness and modulating intercellular junctions. In experimental studies, ROCK inhibitors also reduce extracellular matrix production and fibrosis in trabecular tissues, potentially addressing fundamental pathological changes in glaucomatous eyes.

Netarsudil, the first approved ROCK inhibitor for glaucoma, exhibits a triple mechanism of action: increasing trabecular outflow, decreasing aqueous production (through norepinephrine transporter inhibition), and reducing episcleral venous pressure. This approach provides approximately 16–21% IOP reduction, with efficacy maintained across the full range of baseline pressures. The side effect profile primarily includes conjunctival hyperemia, resulting from ROCK inhibitor-induced vasodilation, and corneal verticillata (asymptomatic corneal deposits) from lysosomally trapped drug metabolites in corneal epithelial cells.

Nitric Oxide Donors: Targeting Conventional Outflow

Latanoprostene bunod represents a novel dual-action compound incorporating a prostaglandin analog moiety (latanoprost acid) with a nitric oxide (NO)-donating group. Upon ocular instillation and corneal esterase activity, this molecule releases both active components, providing complementary mechanisms of IOP reduction.

Nitric oxide functions as a signaling molecule that activates soluble guanylate cyclase, increasing intracellular cyclic guanosine monophosphate (cGMP) levels. In trabecular meshwork cells, elevated cGMP leads to reduced cell contractility, relaxation of the trabecular meshwork, and increased permeability. In Schlemm's canal endothelial cells, NO induces cytoskeletal relaxation and increases the formation of intracellular pores that facilitate aqueous humor drainage. These mechanisms collectively enhance conventional outflow facility beyond that achieved with traditional prostaglandin analogs alone.

The multidimensional approach of targeting both unconventional (via the prostaglandin component) and conventional (via NO donation) outflow pathways provides approximately 1–2 mmHg additional IOP reduction compared to latanoprost alone. The side effect profile remains similar to traditional PGAs, reflecting the conserved prostaglandin structure that mediates most adverse effects.

The diverse mechanisms of action among glaucoma medications provide clinicians with multiple strategies for IOP reduction through complementary physiological pathways. Understanding these mechanisms facilitates rational selection of initial therapy based on individual patient characteristics and informs optimal combination approaches when monotherapy proves insufficient. The continuing development of novel targets, including cytoskeletal modulators, adenosine receptor agonists, and neuroprotective agents, promises to further expand our therapeutic options beyond current IOP-centric approaches, potentially addressing the fundamental neurodegenerative processes underlying glaucomatous optic neuropathy.

Table 5.1 categorizes the major pharmacological agents used in the medical management of glaucoma. It highlights their mechanisms of action, common representatives within each drug class, and typical side effects that clinicians should consider during treatment planning.

Table 5.1 Pharmacological Classes of Anti-Glaucoma Medications

Drug Class	Mechanisms of Action	Common Examples	Typical Side Effects
Prostaglandin Analogues	Increase uveoscleral outflow	Latanoprost, Bimatoprost	Iris pigmentation, eyelash growth
Beta-Blockers	Decrease aqueous production	Timolol, Betaxolol	Bradycardia, hypotension
Alpha-Agonists	Dual action (↓ production, ↑ outflow)	Brimonidine	Allergy, dry mouth
Carbonic Anhydrase Inhibitors	Decrease aqueous production	Dorzolamide, Acetazolamide	Paresthesias, metabolic acidosis (oral)
Rho-Kinase Inhibitors	Increase trabecular outflow	Netarsudil	Conjunctival hyperemia

SECTION 3—CHALLENGES IN PATIENT COMPLIANCE

The effectiveness of glaucoma pharmacotherapy depends not only on the intrinsic efficacy of medications but also critically on patient adherence to prescribed regimens. Despite the availability of potent IOP-lowering agents, suboptimal medication adherence remains a significant barrier to successful glaucoma management. Studies consistently demonstrate that a substantial proportion of patients—ranging from 30% to 80%—fail to use their medications as prescribed. This non-adherence contributes to treatment failure, disease progression, and ultimately, preventable vision loss. This section examines various challenges of patient compliance, methods for assessing adherence, and evidence-based strategies for improving medication-taking behavior in glaucoma patients.

Defining and Measuring Adherence

Medication adherence encompasses multiple related behaviors, including the initial filling of prescriptions (primary adherence), administration of medications at the prescribed frequency and timing (secondary adherence), and persistence with therapy over extended periods. Each component contributes to overall treatment effectiveness and requires specific assessment approaches. Accurately measuring adherence presents significant methodological challenges. Direct methods such as observed therapy or blood level monitoring, though highly accurate, are impractical for chronic glaucoma management. Consequently, research and clinical practice rely on various indirect measures, each with inherent strengths and limitations.

Pharmacy refill data provide objective information about prescription filling patterns without patient awareness that may alter behavior. A study (33) analyzed pharmacy claims data from 13,956 glaucoma patients and found that 37% of patients discontinued all topical glaucoma medications within six months of initial prescription, and 50% had discontinued by two years. This approach, while valuable for population-level analysis, may overestimate actual adherence, as medication possession does not ensure proper administration.

Electronic monitoring devices, considered the current gold standard for research purposes, record the exact date and time of bottle opening, providing detailed patterns of medication use. The Travatan Dosing Aid study (34) used electronic monitors to evaluate adherence patterns in 196 patients over three months, finding that patients took 82% of prescribed doses but administered them within four hours of the scheduled time only 60% of the time. These data highlight the distinction between dose adherence (taking the prescribed number of doses) and timing adherence (taking doses at the correct time)—both essential for optimal IOP control.

Self-reported adherence, typically assessed through questionnaires or interviews, offers practical clinical utility but consistently overestimates actual adherence when compared to objective measures. It was also demonstrated (35) that while 95% of patients self-reported good adherence, electronic monitoring revealed that only 71% actually took more than 75% of prescribed doses. Despite this limitation, self-report measures can identify specific barriers and patterns of non-adherence when administered in a non-judgmental manner.

Factors Affecting Adherence

Medication adherence represents a complex health behavior influenced by multiple interacting factors that extend beyond patient characteristics to include medication properties, provider behaviors, and healthcare system attributes. Demographic factors demonstrate inconsistent associations with adherence. While some studies suggest reduced adherence among younger patients, those of lower socioeconomic status, or certain ethnic minorities, these relationships often diminish when controlling for other variables. More consistent associations emerge with specific patient-centered factors.

Disease knowledge and beliefs significantly impact adherence behavior. In a prospective study (36), it was found that patients with limited understanding of glaucoma's chronicity and potential for blindness demonstrated 2.5 times greater non-adherence compared to those with accurate disease comprehension. Patients who perceive limited benefits from treatment, harbor concerns about medication side effects, or doubt the necessity of treatment in the absence of symptoms typically demonstrate reduced adherence.

Cognitive and functional limitations present substantial barriers to proper medication use. A systematic review (37) identified cognitive impairment, decreased manual dexterity, and physical limitations as significant predictors of non-adherence in elderly glaucoma patients. These factors become particularly relevant considering the aging demographic of the glaucoma population.

Comorbidities and competing health priorities often adversely affect glaucoma medication adherence. Patients managing multiple chronic conditions may prioritize symptomatic conditions over the typically asymptomatic nature of glaucoma. Additionally, polypharmacy increases the complexity of medication regimens, creating challenges for integration of glaucoma medications into daily routines.

Psychological factors, including depression, anxiety, and personality traits, significantly influence adherence behaviors. Depression, prevalent in up to 30% of glaucoma patients, associates with reduced medication adherence across multiple chronic conditions including glaucoma. Another study (38) demonstrated that depressive symptoms correlated with a 1.3-fold increase in non-adherence to glaucoma medications over three years of follow-up, independent of other risk factors.

The properties and characteristics of glaucoma medications themselves significantly influence adherence patterns. Regimen complexity represents one of the most consistently documented barriers to adherence. Studies demonstrate an inverse relationship between dosing frequency and adherence rates, with once-daily regimens achieving approximately 15–20% better adherence than medications requiring administration multiple times daily. Another study (39) found that adherence to once-daily prostaglandin analogs was significantly higher than to twice-daily beta-blockers or three-times-daily alpha-agonists and carbonic anhydrase inhibitors.

Side effects, both symptomatic (hyperemia, burning, stinging) and cosmetic (periorbital fat atrophy, eyelash growth, iris pigmentation), contribute substantially to non-adherence and medication discontinuation. In another study, the authors found that patients experiencing moderate to severe side effects were 2.3 times more likely to discontinue therapy compared to those with mild or no side effects (40).

Medication cost and insurance coverage significantly influence adherence, particularly for patients with limited financial resources. Research (41) has demonstrated that patients with higher copayments were 56% more likely to discontinue prostaglandin analog therapy within the first year compared to those with lower out-of-pocket costs. This cost sensitivity appears particularly pronounced for newer brand-name medications compared to generic alternatives.

Provider communication and the doctor–patient relationship significantly influence adherence behaviors. Studies consistently demonstrate that patients who receive clear, personalized education about their condition and treatment demonstrate better adherence than those receiving standardized or limited information. The quality of the provider–patient relationship, characterized by trust, shared decision-making, and cultural competence, correlates with improved medication adherence and persistence.

Healthcare system barriers, including limited access to care, inadequate insurance coverage, and fragmented care delivery, contribute to reduced adherence rates. Practical challenges such as difficulty obtaining refills, transportation issues, and limited pharmacy hours create additional obstacles to consistent medication use.

Assessment and Monitoring of Adherence in Clinical Practice

Systematically assessing medication adherence in routine clinical practice remains challenging but essential for identifying patients at risk for non-adherence and addressing specific barriers. Several approaches offer practical utility in the clinical setting: Direct questioning about medication use, when posed in a non-judgmental manner, can elicit valuable information about adherence patterns. Questions framed to normalize occasional non-adherence (e.g., "Many people find it difficult to use eye drops regularly. How many doses would you estimate you missed in the past week?") typically yield more accurate responses than accusatory approaches.

Structured questionnaires, including the Glaucoma Treatment Compliance Assessment Tool (GTCAT) and the Morisky Medication Adherence Scale adapted for glaucoma, provide standardized assessment of adherence behaviors and specific barriers. While these instruments demonstrate clinical utility, they should be interpreted recognizing their tendency to overestimate actual adherence.

Clinical markers, including IOP variation between visits, evidence of medication effect (e.g., miosis with pilocarpine), and prescription refill patterns, provide indirect evidence of adherence. While these markers lack sensitivity for detecting moderate non-adherence, significant deviations from expected patterns warrant further exploration of medication-taking behaviors.

Effective interventions to improve medication adherence typically incorporate multiple components tailored to address patient-specific barriers. Several strategies demonstrate evidence of effectiveness in glaucoma management.

Patient education represents a necessary but insufficient component of adherence improvement. A previously mentioned study (35) has demonstrated that an educational intervention consisting of personalized instruction, demonstration, and written materials improved electronically measured adherence from 54% to 73% at three months compared to control subjects. However, this effect diminished over time without additional reinforcement, highlighting the need for ongoing education rather than one-time instruction.

Educational content should address fundamental knowledge gaps regarding the nature of glaucoma as a chronic, progressive condition requiring continuous treatment despite the absence of symptoms. Techniques should incorporate health literacy principles, cultural sensitivity, and adult learning theory to maximize comprehension and retention.

Simplification of medication regimens consistently demonstrates benefit for adherence improvement. When possible, converting from multiple medications to fixed-combination formulations or selecting longer-acting agents requiring less frequent administration (e.g., prostaglandin analogs versus pilocarpine) significantly enhances adherence rates. A study found that simplifying from multiple medications to a fixed combination improved adherence by 23–28% across various chronic conditions including glaucoma (42).

Memory aids and reminders—including medication charts, smartphone applications, and electronic reminder devices—show mixed results when used as isolated interventions but demonstrate greater effectiveness when incorporated into comprehensive programs. A previous study (43) found that automated reminders improved adherence by approximately 11–29% but with considerable heterogeneity in effect size across studies.

Behavioral skills training focuses on developing specific techniques for proper medication administration. This approach includes guided practice of eye drop instillation, strategies for integrating medications into existing daily routines, and problem-solving techniques for managing common barriers. Teaching patients to incorporate medication administration into existing daily habits (habit coupling) appears particularly effective for sustaining long-term adherence.

Involving family members or caregivers in glaucoma management significantly enhances adherence, particularly for elderly patients or those with functional limitations. A study showed that patients with actively engaged family members demonstrated 27% better adherence than those managing medications independently (44). Effective caregiver involvement requires proper education about both the disease and correct medication administration techniques.

Support groups, whether in-person or virtual, provide peer-based encouragement, practical strategies, and normalization of challenges faced by glaucoma patients. While limited research has evaluated their specific impact on medication adherence, qualitative studies suggest they address important psychosocial aspects of chronic disease management that may indirectly support adherence behaviors.

Electronic monitoring devices with adherence feedback provide patients with objective information about their medication-taking patterns, addressing the common disconnect between perceived and actual adherence. A study (45) evaluated a medication alarm device with adherence feedback in 491 glaucoma patients, demonstrating a 16% improvement in adherence compared to controls over nine months of follow-up. Newer "smart" eye drop bottles incorporate usage tracking, automated reminders, and wireless communication capabilities to transmit adherence data to healthcare providers between visits. Emerging evidence suggests these technologies may enhance both adherence and clinical outcomes, though cost considerations currently limit widespread implementation.

Elderly patients with glaucoma face unique adherence challenges including cognitive decline, reduced manual dexterity, and multiple comorbidities. Tailored interventions for this population should emphasize medication organization systems, simplified regimens, engaging caregivers, and assistive devices for eye drop installation. Large-print instructions with visual cues rather than text-heavy materials better accommodate age-related visual and cognitive changes.

Patients with low health literacy require specific approaches to enhance understanding and adherence. Educational materials should utilize plain language, incorporate visual aids, employ the teach-back method to confirm comprehension, and avoid medical jargon. Existing research demonstrated that a health literacy-focused educational program improved adherence by 16% compared to standard care among glaucoma patients with limited health literacy (46).

Optimizing adherence to glaucoma medications requires a special approach that addresses the complex interplay of patient, medication, provider, and healthcare system factors influencing medication-taking behaviors. Effective management strategies incorporate assessment of individual adherence patterns and barriers, followed by tailored interventions that may include education, behavioral strategies, social support, and technological assistance. By systematically addressing adherence as a fundamental component of glaucoma management rather than an assumed behavior, clinicians can enhance treatment effectiveness, improve clinical outcomes, and ultimately preserve vision for patients with this chronic, progressive disease.

CHAPTER 6
SURGICAL AND LASER TREATMENTS

While pharmacological therapy remains the initial approach for most glaucoma patients, surgical and laser interventions play a critical role in the comprehensive management of this potentially blinding disease. The evolution of glaucoma surgery represents one of the most dynamic areas in ophthalmology, with significant innovations expanding the therapeutic options available to surgeons and patients alike. Modern glaucoma surgery encompasses a spectrum of procedures ranging from traditional filtering operations to micro-invasive approaches, each offering distinct risk–benefit profiles that must be carefully considered when developing individualized treatment strategies.

The fundamental goal of glaucoma surgery remains consistent—to reduce intraocular pressure to a level that prevents further optic nerve damage while minimizing complications and preserving visual function. However, the means of achieving this goal have diversified substantially. Traditional filtering procedures such as trabeculectomy create an alternative pathway for aqueous humor outflow through a guarded fistula between the anterior chamber and subconjunctival space. These procedures, while highly effective at lowering intraocular pressure, carry significant risks including hypotony, infection, and bleb-related complications. Nonetheless, they remain essential options for patients with advanced or rapidly progressive disease requiring substantial pressure reduction.

The past two decades have witnessed a revolutionary expansion of the surgical armamentarium with the development of minimally invasive glaucoma surgery (MIGS). These procedures aim to enhance conventional physiologic outflow pathways while minimizing tissue disruption and risk. By offering modest but clinically meaningful pressure reduction with enhanced safety profiles, MIGS has fundamentally altered the risk–benefit calculus of glaucoma surgery, potentially lowering the threshold for earlier surgical intervention in the disease course. Laser treatments occupy a unique position in the glaucoma treatment paradigm, offering non-incisional approaches that can be performed in outpatient settings with rapid recovery. From selective laser trabeculoplasty to laser peripheral iridotomy and cyclophotocoagulation, these modalities provide important options that may delay or reduce the need for more invasive interventions or topical medications.

This chapter explores the full spectrum of contemporary surgical and laser approaches to glaucoma management, examining the technical aspects, indications, outcomes, and complications of each procedure type. By understanding the relative advantages and limitations of these various interventions, clinicians can develop optimally tailored treatment strategies for individual patients based on disease severity, progression rate, risk factors, and personal preferences.

DOI: 10.1201/9781003646693-6

SECTION I—TRADITIONAL SURGERIES: TRABECULECTOMY AND BEYOND

Traditional glaucoma surgeries have formed the foundation of surgical management for decades, providing substantial intraocular pressure (IOP) reduction for patients with moderate to advanced disease or those progressing despite maximal medical therapy. These procedures create alternative pathways for aqueous humor outflow, bypassing the compromised conventional outflow system. While associated with higher complication rates than newer minimally invasive approaches, traditional surgeries remain essential options in the glaucoma treatment paradigm, particularly for patients requiring substantial pressure reduction or those with advanced disease. This section examines the principles, techniques, outcomes, and complications of these established surgical interventions.

Trabeculectomy: The Gold Standard

Since its introduction by Cairns in 1968, trabeculectomy has remained the most commonly performed incisional glaucoma procedure worldwide. The surgery creates a guarded fistula between the anterior chamber and the subconjunctival space, establishing an alternative pathway for aqueous outflow. The basic technique involves creating a partial-thickness scleral flap, excising a portion of the trabecular meshwork and adjacent structures to access the anterior chamber, and suturing the scleral flap to provide controlled aqueous outflow. The overlying conjunctiva forms a filtering bleb that collects and absorbs the diverted aqueous humor.

While numerous modifications exist, the core technique involves several key steps: Conjunctival dissection (either limbus- or fornix-based), creation of a partial-thickness scleral flap (typically rectangular or triangular), application of an antimetabolite to reduce scarring, excision of a trabecular tissue block, peripheral iridectomy to prevent iris blockage of the sclerostomy, and careful closure of the scleral flap and conjunctiva. The degree of flap tension, determined by the number and tightness of scleral flap sutures, represents a critical factor in determining immediate postoperative IOP.

Modern trabeculectomy incorporates several refinements that have improved outcomes and reduced complications. Antimetabolites, particularly mitomycin C (MMC) and 5-fluorouracil (5-FU), have dramatically enhanced success rates by modulating wound healing and reducing scarring. A landmark study by the Fluorouracil Filtering Surgery Study Group (47) demonstrated significantly improved surgical outcomes with adjunctive 5-FU in high-risk patients, establishing antimetabolites as a standard component of modern trabeculectomy. Contemporary surgeons typically apply MMC (0.2–0.4 mg/mL) for 1–4 minutes intraoperatively, with concentration and exposure time tailored to the patient's risk profile for scarring.

Releasable or adjustable sutures provide enhanced control of early postoperative filtration, allowing the surgeon to titrate flow gradually as healing progresses, thereby reducing risks of hypotony while maintaining filtration. Laser suture lysis offers an alternative approach to adjusting flow in the early postoperative period.

Trabeculectomy demonstrates substantial efficacy in lowering IOP, typically achieving pressures in the low-to-mid teens and reductions of 30–50% from baseline. The tube versus trabeculectomy (TVT) study, a multicenter randomized clinical trial comparing trabeculectomy with tube shunt surgery in patients with previous ocular surgery or failed trabeculectomy, reported mean IOP reduction from 25.6 mmHg to 13.5 mmHg at one year and 14.4 mmHg at five years in the trabeculectomy group (48). This robust pressure-lowering effect often allows reduction or elimination of glaucoma medications, with 63% of trabeculectomy patients requiring no supplemental medication at five years in the TVT study.

Success rates vary by definition criteria, follow-up duration, patient population, and surgical technique. Contemporary studies with strict success definitions (including upper and lower IOP limits) typically report qualified success rates (with or without medications) of 70–90% at one year, declining to 50–70% at five years. Factors affecting success include patient age, race, glaucoma type, previous surgery, and postoperative management. African American race, younger age, previous surgery, and certain secondary glaucomas (particularly neovascular and uveitic) associate with higher failure rates due to more aggressive healing responses.

Despite its efficacy, trabeculectomy carries significant risks that must be carefully considered when selecting surgical candidates. Early complications include hypotony (potentially resulting in choroidal effusion, suprachoroidal hemorrhage, or hypotony maculopathy), shallow or flat anterior chamber, hyphema, and aqueous misdirection syndrome. Late complications include bleb leak, bleb encapsulation, bleb-related infection (ranging from blebitis to endophthalmitis), and cataract progression.

Bleb-related infection represents one of the most serious complications, with reported rates of bleb-related endophthalmitis ranging from 0.2–1.5% per patient-year with MMC-augmented procedures. Risk factors include inferiorly positioned blebs, thin avascular blebs, bleb leaks, blepharitis, and younger patient age. The risk-benefit profile of trabeculectomy necessitates careful patient selection and informed consent discussions highlighting both the substantial pressure-lowering benefit and the significant potential complications.

Glaucoma Drainage Devices

Glaucoma drainage devices (GDDs), also known as tube shunts or aqueous shunts, represent important alternatives to trabeculectomy, particularly in cases with high risk for trabeculectomy failure. These devices divert aqueous humor from the anterior chamber to an equatorial plate positioned beneath the conjunctiva and Tenon's capsule, where a fibrous capsule forms to regulate flow and absorption.

GDDs are categorized as either valved (Ahmed) or non-valved (Baerveldt, Molteno) implants. Valved devices incorporate flow-restriction mechanisms designed to prevent early postoperative hypotony, allowing immediate flow while theoretically maintaining pressures above a threshold (typically 8–10 mmHg). Non-valved implants require temporary flow restriction, typically with an external ligature that dissolves or is removed postoperatively, or an internal occluding stent that is later removed or fenestrated.

Device selection considers factors including surgeon familiarity, target IOP, hypotony risk, and prior surgical history. Plate size (ranging from 96–350 mm²) influences final IOP, with larger plates generally associated with lower long-term pressures but increased risk of diplopia and motility disturbances.

Standard GDD implantation involves conjunctival dissection to expose the intended plate position (typically superotemporal), secure fixation of the plate to underlying sclera, creation of a tunnel for the tube from the plate to limbus, insertion of the tube into the anterior chamber through a needle tract, and careful coverage of the exposed tube with patch graft material (preserved sclera, pericardium, or cornea) to prevent erosion. For non-valved implants, temporary tube ligation using absorbable suture with or without a venting incision controls early postoperative flow.

The tube versus trabeculectomy study provided robust comparative data between these approaches. At five years, mean IOP was similar between groups (14.4 mmHg in trabeculectomy vs. 14.5 mmHg in tube group), but the tube group required more medications (2.1 vs. 1.2). The cumulative probability of failure was higher with trabeculectomy (46.9% vs. 29.8%), primarily due to persistent hypotony and bleb-related complications. Early postoperative complications occurred more frequently with trabeculectomy, though late complications and serious complications were similar between groups.

The primary tube versus trabeculectomy (PTVT) study examined these surgeries in patients without previous incisional ocular surgery, addressing a critical knowledge gap regarding their comparative efficacy as primary surgical interventions. Initial reports suggest similar IOP reduction with fewer complications in the tube group, though complete long-term results are forthcoming.

Nonpenetrating Glaucoma Surgery

Nonpenetrating procedures, including deep sclerectomy and viscocanalostomy, were developed to enhance safety by avoiding full-thickness penetration into the anterior chamber, theoretically reducing complications associated with sudden decompression and aqueous overfiltration.

Deep sclerectomy involves creating a deep scleral flap, dissecting a second deeper flap to expose Descemet's membrane (creating the "scleral lake"), unroofing Schlemm's canal, and removing the inner wall of Schlemm's canal and juxtacanalicular trabecular meshwork. This establishes a permeable membrane through which aqueous can percolate without the rapid decompression associated with penetrating procedures. Implantation of space-maintaining devices (collagen, hyaluronic acid, or acrylic implants) or application of antimetabolites may enhance long-term outcomes.

Viscocanalostomy similarly creates a deep scleral lake but focuses on dilating Schlemm's canal with viscoelastic to enhance conventional outflow. The procedure does not rely on external filtration but rather aims to enhance physiologic outflow pathways.

Studies comparing these nonpenetrating approaches with trabeculectomy generally demonstrate more modest IOP reduction with nonpenetrating procedures but fewer complications, particularly those related to hypotony. A meta-analysis (49) found that while trabeculectomy achieved lower mean IOP, nonpenetrating surgeries had significantly lower risks of hypotony, choroidal detachment, and cataract progression. The technical difficulty of nonpenetrating procedures, combined with the frequent need for subsequent goniopuncture to enhance flow through the trabeculo-Descemet's membrane, has limited their widespread adoption, particularly in North America.

Cyclodestructive Procedures

Cyclodestructive procedures reduce aqueous production by ablating portions of the ciliary body epithelium responsible for aqueous secretion. While traditionally reserved for refractory glaucoma or eyes with limited visual potential, refinements in technique and delivery have expanded their application.

Transscleral cyclophotocoagulation (CPC) applies diode laser energy through the sclera to the underlying ciliary body, typically treating 180–270 degrees in a single session. Newer approaches employ micropulse delivery to potentially reduce inflammation and collateral tissue damage. Endoscopic cyclophotocoagulation (ECP) provides direct visualization of the ciliary processes through an intraocular approach, allowing more precise treatment with potentially fewer complications than transscleral approaches.

While historically associated with significant complications including vision loss, hypotony, and phthisis bulbi, modern techniques with titrated treatment energy and extent have substantially improved the safety profile of these procedures, leading some surgeons to utilize them earlier in the treatment algorithm, particularly in patients at high risk for filtering surgery complications.

To conclude this section, traditional glaucoma surgeries continue to play a vital role in the surgical management of glaucoma, particularly for patients with advanced disease, requiring substantial pressure reduction, or at high risk for progression. While newer minimally invasive approaches have expanded the surgical armamentarium, procedures such as trabeculectomy and tube shunt implantation remain essential options offering powerful IOP reduction. The ongoing refinement of these techniques, coupled with improved understanding of wound healing modulation and postoperative management, has enhanced outcomes while specific patient factors and risk profiles continue to guide appropriate procedure selection in the era of personalized glaucoma care.

SECTION 2—MINIMALLY INVASIVE GLAUCOMA SURGERIES (MIGS)

The emergence of minimally invasive glaucoma surgeries (MIGS) represents one of the most significant paradigm shifts in glaucoma management over the past two decades. These procedures aim to provide a more favorable safety profile than traditional filtering surgeries while offering modest but clinically meaningful reductions in intraocular pressure (IOP) and medication burden. The MIGS revolution has been driven by the recognition that many patients, particularly those with mild to moderate disease, require an intervention that bridges the gap between medications and more invasive traditional surgeries. This section examines the diverse array of MIGS procedures, their mechanisms of action, surgical techniques, efficacy profiles, and appropriate patient selection criteria.

While no universally accepted definition exists, MIGS procedures generally share several key characteristics: ab interno approach (though some newer procedures utilize ab externo techniques), minimal conjunctival manipulation, minimal scleral dissection, and rapid recovery with minimal impact on refractive outcomes. These procedures typically demonstrate a high safety profile with limited sight-threatening complications, though they generally provide more modest IOP reduction compared to traditional filtering surgeries.

MIGS procedures can be classified by their anatomical target and mechanism of action:

1. *Trabecular Meshwork Bypass/Excision*: Procedures that bypass or remove the trabecular meshwork to enhance conventional outflow through Schlemm's canal and collector channels (e.g., iStent, Hydrus, Trabectome, Kahook Dual Blade, GATT)
2. *Subconjunctival Filtration*: Procedures that create a controlled subconjunctival filtration pathway (e.g., XEN Gel Stent, PRESERFLO MicroShunt)
3. *Suprachoroidal Shunting*: Devices that enhance uveoscleral outflow by creating a connection between the anterior chamber and the suprachoroidal space (e.g., CyPass Micro-Stent [withdrawn from market])
4. *Ciliary Process Ablation*: Procedures that reduce aqueous production through targeted treatment of the ciliary processes (e.g., Endoscopic Cyclophotocoagulation)

This classification system helps conceptualize the various approaches and their expected effects on aqueous dynamics.

Trabecular Meshwork Bypass/Excision Procedures

Trabecular Micro-Bypass Stents

The iStent (Glaukos Corporation) became the first FDA-approved MIGS device in 2012, pioneering the category. This heparin-coated, non-ferromagnetic titanium device is inserted through the trabecular meshwork into Schlemm's canal, creating a direct pathway for aqueous to bypass the trabecular resistance. Multiple generations of the device have been developed, including the first-generation iStent, iStent Inject (which includes two smaller stents), and iStent Infinite (a three-stent system). Clinical studies demonstrate modest efficacy when combined with cataract surgery. A landmark randomized controlled trial (50) comparing cataract surgery alone versus cataract surgery with iStent implantation showed that 72% of combination patients versus 50% of cataract-only patients achieved an IOP ≤21 mmHg without medications at one year. The iStent Inject, with its two-stent design potentially accessing more collector channels, demonstrated slightly improved efficacy in subsequent studies.

The Hydrus Microstent (Ivantis Inc.) represents an evolution in trabecular micro-bypass technology, featuring an 8 mm scaffold that dilates and maintains patency of Schlemm's canal while also providing direct trabecular bypass. The HORIZON study, a multicenter randomized controlled trial comparing cataract surgery alone versus cataract surgery with Hydrus implantation, demonstrated that at 24 months, 73% of Hydrus patients versus 48% of control patients were medication-free, with the treatment group also showing lower mean IOP (17.4 mmHg vs. 19.2 mmHg). The unique design of the Hydrus, which spans approximately 3 clock hours of Schlemm's canal, may provide access to more collector channels than point-bypass devices.

Both trabecular micro-bypass technologies demonstrate excellent safety profiles with few serious complications. Mild hyphema is the most common intraoperative complication, typically resolving within days. Rare complications include device malposition, obstruction, or corneal endothelial cell loss. The favorable risk profile makes these devices particularly appropriate for patients with mild to moderate open-angle glaucoma undergoing cataract surgery.

Trabecular Ablation/Excision

Procedures that ablate or excise the trabecular meshwork offer the potential advantage of treating a broader area of outflow resistance compared to focal stent placement. These approaches include the Trabectome (NeoMedix Corporation), which uses electrocautery to ablate a strip of trabecular meshwork and inner wall of Schlemm's canal, and the Kahook Dual Blade (New World Medical), which precisely excises a strip of trabecular meshwork while preserving adjacent tissue.

Studies of the Trabectome demonstrate mean IOP reductions of approximately 30–40% with a reduction in medications when performed as a standalone procedure. When combined with cataract surgery, slightly greater IOP reductions may be achieved. The Kahook Dual Blade demonstrates similar efficacy, with mean IOP reductions of 24–26% in standalone procedures and slightly greater reductions when combined with cataract surgery. These procedures involve direct visualization using a gonioprism, minimal conjunctival manipulation, and rapid recovery. Complications are generally limited to intraoperative bleeding, transient IOP elevation, and potential need for secondary procedures if the treatment effect diminishes over time.

Gonioscopy-Assisted Transluminal Trabeculotomy (GATT)

GATT represents an innovative adaptation of traditional external trabeculotomy to an ab interno, minimally invasive approach. The procedure involves creating a small goniotomy incision in the trabecular meshwork, then using a microcatheter or suture to cannulate Schlemm's canal for 360 degrees before externalizing the distal end, creating a complete circumferential trabeculotomy. This technique opens the entire trabecular outflow system rather than focusing on focal bypass or excision. GATT procedure has demonstrated promising results across various glaucoma types. In their initial report of 85 eyes with open-angle glaucoma, Grover and colleagues found mean IOP reduction from 24.7 mmHg to 15.7 mmHg at 12 months in primary open-angle glaucoma cases, with medication reduction from 3.2 to 1.5 medications. Even more impressive results were noted in patients with secondary open-angle glaucoma. GATT offers several advantages: It can be performed through a small clear corneal incision, requires no conjunctival dissection, preserves conjunctival tissue for future procedures if needed, and addresses the entire trabecular outflow system. The procedure has expanded from adult open-angle glaucoma to include pediatric glaucoma, angle-closure glaucoma following iridotomy, and various secondary glaucomas.

Complications include transient hyphema (nearly universal but typically resolving within 1–2 weeks), early IOP spikes (usually responsive to medical management), and occasional failure to complete the 360-degree catheterization due to anatomical obstructions. Rarely, Descemet detachment or iris prolapse may occur. Despite these potential complications, the procedure demonstrates an overall favorable safety profile compared to traditional filtering surgeries.

Subconjunctival Filtration Devices

XEN Gel Stent

The XEN Gel Stent (Allergan, an AbbVie company) represents a novel approach that combines elements of traditional filtering surgery with minimally invasive technique. This 6 mm hydrophilic gelatin stent creates a subconjunctival filtration pathway, conceptually similar to trabeculectomy but delivered through an ab interno approach that spares conjunctival dissection.

The procedure involves inserting the preloaded stent through a clear corneal incision, across the anterior chamber, and through the angle to create a connection between the anterior chamber and subconjunctival space. Adjunctive mitomycin C is typically used to reduce scarring and improve long-term outcomes. This approach creates a filtering bleb similar to trabeculectomy but through a less invasive surgical approach. Clinical studies demonstrate significant IOP-lowering efficacy, with mean reductions of approximately 30–40% from baseline and substantial decreases in medication use. A prospective study (51) reported mean IOP reduction from 20.0 mmHg to 13.9 mmHg at two years, with medication reduction from 2.4 to 0.4 medications. While the XEN procedure avoids conjunctival dissection, complications similar to traditional filtering surgery can occur, including hypotony, choroidal effusion, bleb-related complications (leaks, fibrosis), and rarely, endophthalmitis. Post-operative bleb management, including potential needling procedures to address fibrosis, represents an important aspect of long-term care. The safety profile falls between trabecular MIGS and traditional trabeculectomy, positioning the XEN as an option for moderate to advanced glaucoma patients requiring greater pressure reduction than typically achieved with trabecular procedures.

PRESERFLO MicroShunt

The PRESERFLO MicroShunt (formerly InnFocus MicroShunt, Santen Pharmaceutical) utilizes an ab externo approach with a flexible, biocompatible, flow-restricting tube that shunts aqueous from the anterior chamber to the subconjunctival space. While requiring conjunctival dissection, the procedure is less invasive than traditional trabeculectomy and creates a posterior filtration bleb designed to reduce bleb-related complications. Early clinical studies have shown promising results, with IOP reductions comparable to trabeculectomy but with potentially fewer complications. The device design incorporates flow restriction to reduce hypotony risk while providing substantial pressure reduction for patients with more advanced disease or requiring lower target pressures.

Ciliary Process Procedures

Endoscopic Cyclophotocoagulation (ECP)

ECP selectively treats ciliary processes under direct endoscopic visualization to reduce aqueous production. This targeted approach differs from traditional transscleral cyclophotocoagulation by allowing precise treatment of selected ciliary processes while minimizing collateral tissue damage. The procedure involves introducing an endoscopic probe through a clear corneal incision, allowing visualization and selective laser ablation of the ciliary processes. When combined with cataract surgery, ECP demonstrates IOP reductions of 15–30% from baseline with reduced medication requirements. Standalone ECP may offer similar or slightly more modest results depending on the extent of treatment. Complications are generally less severe than with transscleral cyclophotocoagulation and include transient inflammation, pressure spikes, cystoid macular edema, and rarely, hypotony or phthisis. The direct visualization aspect significantly enhances safety compared to external cyclodestructive procedures.

Patient Selection and Procedure Choice

Appropriate patient selection is critical for optimizing MIGS outcomes. Several factors guide procedure selection.

- *Disease severity and target IOP*: Trabecular procedures typically achieve final IOPs in the mid-to-high teens and are most appropriate for mild to moderate disease. Subconjunctival approaches can achieve lower target pressures (low-to-mid teens) and may be more suitable for advanced disease or patients requiring lower target pressures.
- *Angle anatomy*: Trabecular procedures require adequate angle visualization and access to the trabecular meshwork. Narrow angles or extensive peripheral anterior synechiae may preclude certain trabecular approaches.
- *Prior conjunctival surgery*: Previous conjunctival surgery may influence procedure selection, potentially favoring trabecular or endoscopic approaches that spare the conjunctiva for patients with extensive conjunctival scarring.
- *Medication tolerance*: Patients with ocular surface disease or compliance challenges may particularly benefit from MIGS to reduce medication burden, even when IOP is controlled medically.
- *Concurrent cataract surgery*: Many MIGS procedures demonstrate enhanced efficacy and cost-effectiveness when combined with cataract surgery, influencing timing and procedure selection.

In conclusion, the MIGS revolution has fundamentally altered the glaucoma treatment paradigm, offering intermediate options between medical therapy and traditional incisional surgery. These procedures demonstrate substantial heterogeneity in approach, efficacy, and safety profiles, allowing tailored selection based on individual patient characteristics and treatment goals. While generally providing more modest IOP reduction than traditional filtering surgery, their enhanced safety profile and rapid recovery have expanded the population of patients for whom surgical intervention may be appropriate. As long-term data accumulate and new technologies emerge, the role of MIGS in glaucoma management continues to evolve, with increasing potential for earlier surgical intervention in the disease process.

SECTION 3—ROLE OF LASER THERAPY IN MODERN PRACTICE

Laser therapies occupy a unique position in the glaucoma treatment paradigm, offering non-incisional intervention options with substantial efficacy and generally favorable safety profiles. These procedures can be performed in outpatient settings with minimal recovery time, avoid the complications associated with invasive surgery, and preserve the conjunctiva for future interventions if needed. As the glaucoma management landscape evolves, laser therapies continue to demonstrate important roles both as initial interventions and as adjunctive treatments throughout the disease course. This section examines the major laser modalities used in contemporary glaucoma practice, their mechanisms of action, efficacy profiles, and appropriate clinical applications.

Laser Trabeculoplasty

Laser trabeculoplasty enhances aqueous outflow by applying laser energy to the trabecular meshwork, improving conventional outflow facility. Since its introduction in the 1970s, this approach has evolved through several iterations with refinements in laser technology and application parameters.

Selective Laser Trabeculoplasty (SLT)

SLT has largely supplanted earlier argon laser trabeculoplasty (ALT) techniques in contemporary practice. SLT employs a Q-switched, frequency-doubled Nd:YAG laser (532 nm) that selectively targets pigmented trabecular meshwork cells without causing coagulative damage to adjacent non-pigmented structures or the trabecular beams. This selective photothermolysis mechanism differs fundamentally from the non-selective thermal damage induced by ALT.

The procedure typically involves applying 50–100 confluent but non-overlapping laser spots over 180–360 degrees of the trabecular meshwork using a goniolens. The selective nature of SLT allows for repeated treatments, unlike ALT which causes more permanent structural alterations that limit retreatment potential.

The cellular and molecular mechanisms underlying SLT efficacy remain incompletely understood but likely involve multiple pathways. The selective targeting of pigmented trabecular meshwork cells triggers a cascade of biological responses including cytokine release, matrix metalloproteinase induction, macrophage recruitment, and remodeling of the extracellular matrix. These changes collectively enhance aqueous outflow facility without the scarring associated with non-selective laser techniques.

The laser in glaucoma and ocular hypertension (LiGHT) trial, a landmark multicenter randomized controlled trial, compared SLT with topical medication as initial therapy for open-angle glaucoma and ocular hypertension. At 36 months, it was reported (14) that 74.2% of SLT patients required no drops to maintain target IOP, with similar IOP control between groups but fewer glaucoma surgeries required in the SLT arm (0 vs. 11). Based on these compelling results, SLT is increasingly positioned as a viable first-line treatment option rather than simply an alternative after medication failure.

Clinical efficacy of SLT demonstrates considerable variability between patients. Overall, mean IOP reductions of 20–30% can be expected, with response rates (defined as ≥20% IOP reduction) of 60–80%. Factors associated with favorable response include higher baseline IOP, greater angle pigmentation, and pseudoexfoliation glaucoma. Efficacy tends to diminish over time, with approximately 50% of initially successful treatments maintaining efficacy at two years and further declines thereafter, though retreatment can often restore the therapeutic effect. Complications of SLT are generally mild and transient. Approximately 5–10% of patients experience an IOP spike, which typically resolves within 24 hours with or without additional medication. Mild anterior chamber inflammation occurs frequently but seldom causes symptoms and generally resolves without intervention within 1–5 days. Rare complications include corneal edema, hyphema, and persistent IOP elevation.

Micropulse Laser Trabeculoplasty (MLT)

Micropulse laser trabeculoplasty represents a newer approach that delivers laser energy in short pulses separated by rest periods, theoretically reducing collateral thermal damage. The technique utilizes an 810 nm diode laser with energy delivered in microsecond pulses, allowing tissue cooling between pulses. This approach may further reduce inflammatory response and tissue damage compared to conventional continuous-wave lasers. Early studies suggest efficacy comparable to SLT with potentially fewer side effects, though long-term comparative data remain limited. The mechanism likely involves similar biological responses to SLT with subtle differences related to the thermal relaxation characteristics of the micropulse delivery.

Laser Peripheral Iridotomy (LPI)

Laser peripheral iridotomy creates a full-thickness opening in the peripheral iris to equalize pressure between the anterior and posterior chambers, thereby eliminating pupillary block and allowing the iris to fall back from the angle. This procedure represents the definitive treatment for pupillary block and the cornerstone of angle-closure management. The procedure is typically performed using a Nd:YAG laser, though a sequential argon-YAG technique may be employed for thicker, more pigmented irides. The iridotomy site is usually positioned in the superior iris (between 10 and 2 o'clock) where it will be covered by the upper eyelid, minimizing dysphotopsia symptoms. The size of the iridotomy should be at least 150–200 μm to prevent closure. In primary angle-closure suspect (PACS) and primary angle-closure (PAC), LPI effectively eliminates pupillary block, deepens the anterior chamber, and widens the angle in the majority of cases. However, in primary angle-closure glaucoma (PACG) with established optic neuropathy, additional IOP-lowering interventions are frequently required despite successful anatomical correction of pupillary block. The role of prophylactic LPI in angle-closure suspects has evolved with emerging evidence. The ZAP (Zhongshan angle closure prevention) trial, a landmark randomized controlled trial involving 889 Chinese participants with bilateral PACS, found that prophylactic LPI reduced the incidence of angle-closure disease from 4.19% to 2.35% over six years of follow-up. However, this modest absolute risk reduction of 1.84% has prompted more selective approaches to prophylactic treatment, particularly in populations with lower baseline risk. Complications of LPI include transient IOP elevation (10–15% of cases), bleeding from the iris (common but rarely significant), corneal endothelial burns, posterior synechiae, and rarely, cataract formation if the lens is inadvertently damaged. Visual symptoms including monocular diplopia, ghosting, or glare may occur in 10–15% of patients despite superior placement.

Laser Iridoplasty

Peripheral laser iridoplasty applies low-energy, long-duration burns to the peripheral iris to contract the iris stroma, pulling the peripheral iris away from the angle. This procedure addresses plateau iris syndrome and other non-pupillary block mechanisms of angle closure that persist after successful iridotomy. The technique employs an argon laser with large spot size (500 μm), low power (200–400 mW), and long duration (0.5 seconds), creating contraction burns rather than penetrating the iris. Multiple spots are placed circumferentially in the far peripheral iris to achieve maximal widening of the angle. Clinical indications include persistent appositional angle closure after successful LPI, plateau iris syndrome, and occasionally as a temporizing measure in acute angle closure when immediate LPI is technically challenging. While effective in the short term, the effect may diminish over time, and iridoplasty does not address the fundamental anatomical configuration of plateau iris syndrome.

Cyclophotocoagulation

Cyclophotocoagulation (CPC) reduces aqueous production by thermally ablating ciliary body epithelium. Traditional transscleral CPC has evolved from a procedure reserved for end-stage, refractory glaucoma to a more precisely titrated intervention applicable earlier in the disease course for selected patients.

Transscleral Cyclophotocoagulation

Transsceral CPC delivers diode laser energy (810 nm) through the sclera to the underlying ciliary body, typically treating 180–270 degrees of the ciliary body in a single session. Energy settings and treatment extent are tailored to the clinical scenario, with more conservative approaches for eyes with better visual potential. The procedure can be performed using either a contact G-probe that positions the laser energy 1.2 mm posterior to the limbus or with a non-contact delivery system. While historically associated with significant complications including vision loss, hypotony, and phthisis bulbi, modern protocol refinements with reduced energy settings have substantially improved the safety profile.

Micropulse Transsceral Cyclophotocoagulation (MP-TSCPC)

Micropulse TSCPC delivers energy in short pulses separated by rest periods, theoretically allowing for tissue cooling and reduced collateral damage. Early studies suggest this approach may offer comparable IOP reduction to conventional CPC with lower complication rates, potentially expanding the applications of cyclophotocoagulation to earlier-stage glaucoma. An exploratory study (52) demonstrated similar IOP-lowering efficacy between continuous and micropulse delivery, but with significantly lower complication rates in the micropulse group.

Endoscopic Cyclophotocoagulation (ECP)

As discussed in the MIGS section, ECP provides direct visualization of the ciliary processes, allowing targeted and precise treatment while minimizing collateral damage. This approach represents a significant evolution from traditional transscleral techniques and is increasingly incorporated into combined cataract-glaucoma surgical plans.

Integration of Laser Therapies in the Treatment Algorithm

The positioning of laser therapies within the glaucoma treatment algorithm continues to evolve based on emerging evidence. Several important trends and considerations influence contemporary practice:

- *SLT as initial therapy*: The LiGHT trial has provided strong evidence supporting SLT as a viable first-line option, particularly for patients with adherence concerns, tolerability issues with medications, or preference for a drop-free initial approach. Cost-effectiveness analyses generally favor this approach when considering lifetime treatment costs and quality of life impacts.
- *Selective application of prophylactic LPI*: Evidence from the ZAP trial suggests a more selective approach to prophylactic LPI for primary angle-closure suspects, potentially targeting higher-risk individuals rather than universal treatment of all anatomically narrow angles.
- *Expanded applications of cyclophotocoagulation*: With refinements in technique and delivery, particularly micropulse technology, cyclophotocoagulation is

increasingly considered for cases beyond end-stage refractory glaucoma, though patient selection remains critical.

- *Laser as bridge therapy*: Laser interventions (particularly SLT and MP-TSCPC) can serve as valuable temporizing measures for patients awaiting more definitive surgical intervention or for whom surgery carries excessive risk.
- *Combination approaches*: Sequential or simultaneous application of multiple laser modalities (e.g., SLT following LPI in mixed-mechanism glaucoma) may address multiple aspects of outflow dysfunction in complex cases.

Evidently, laser therapies offer important non-incisional options throughout the glaucoma disease spectrum, from primary intervention to adjunctive therapy in advanced disease. Their favorable safety profiles, outpatient delivery, and conjunctival-sparing nature provide significant advantages in the treatment algorithm. As technology continues to evolve, particularly with micropulse delivery systems and refined treatment parameters, the applications and positioning of laser therapy will likely continue to expand, further enhancing the glaucoma specialist's armamentarium in addressing this complex disease.

CHAPTER 7
ADVANCES IN GLAUCOMA RESEARCH

The landscape of glaucoma management is undergoing a remarkable transformation, driven by unprecedented scientific and technological advancements that promise to revolutionize how we diagnose, monitor, and treat this complex disease. As our understanding of glaucoma pathophysiology deepens and technology continues to evolve at an accelerating pace, the potential for fundamental paradigm shifts in glaucoma care has never been greater. This chapter explores the cutting-edge innovations and emerging approaches that are reshaping the field and offering new hope for improved patient outcomes.

The historical conceptualization of glaucoma as simply an "elevated pressure disease" has given way to recognition of its multifactorial nature involving complex interactions among vascular, biomechanical, immunological, and neurodegenerative mechanisms. This expanded understanding has catalyzed research across multiple disciplines, from molecular biology to biomedical engineering, artificial intelligence, and precision medicine. The convergence of these fields is generating novel approaches that address not only intraocular pressure but also the fundamental neuroprotection and even neuroregeneration that represent the ultimate goals of treatment.

In this chapter, we first examine innovations in diagnostic technology that are enhancing our ability to detect glaucoma earlier and monitor progression with unprecedented precision. From advanced imaging modalities to home-monitoring devices and artificial intelligence applications, these tools promise more personalized and effective disease management. We then explore experimental therapeutic approaches, including neuroprotection strategies, gene therapy, stem cell applications, and novel drug delivery systems that may fundamentally alter treatment paradigms. Finally, we examine future directions in glaucoma care, including the integration of big data and artificial intelligence into clinical decision-making, teleophthalmology applications, and the potential for precision medicine approaches tailored to individual risk profiles and disease mechanisms.

While many of these innovations remain in developmental or early clinical stages, their collective potential suggests a future where glaucoma diagnosis occurs before functional damage, treatment addresses fundamental neuropathological mechanisms, and visual impairment becomes increasingly preventable through personalized interventions throughout the disease course.

DOI: 10.1201/9781003646693-7

SECTION I—INNOVATIONS IN DIAGNOSTIC TOOLS

The early detection and accurate monitoring of glaucoma remain fundamental challenges in ophthalmology. Despite significant advances in understanding the disease, glaucoma continues to be diagnosed after substantial irreversible damage has already occurred, with an estimated 50–60% of retinal ganglion cells lost before conventional visual field defects become detectable. This diagnostic gap has driven intensive research into novel technologies aimed at earlier detection, more precise characterization, and more sensitive progression monitoring. This section explores cutting-edge diagnostic innovations that promise to transform glaucoma care from reactive management to proactive intervention.

Advanced Imaging Technologies

Optical Coherence Tomography Angiography (OCTA)

Optical coherence tomography angiography represents one of the most significant recent advances in ophthalmic imaging. This noninvasive technology provides three-dimensional visualization of the retinal and optic nerve head vasculature without requiring intravenous contrast injection. By detecting temporal changes in OCT signals caused by moving blood cells, OCTA generates detailed maps of microvascular networks in various retinal layers and the optic nerve head. In glaucoma, OCTA has revealed significant vascular alterations that may precede structural neural tissue loss. Studies have demonstrated reduced vessel density in the peripapillary retina, optic nerve head, and macula in glaucomatous eyes compared to healthy controls. A comprehensive analysis (53) found that peripapillary OCTA vessel density measurements showed diagnostic accuracy comparable to RNFL thickness measurements for differentiating between glaucomatous and normal eyes, with areas under the receiver operating characteristic curve of 0.94 and 0.95, respectively. Particularly promising is the potential for OCTA to detect early disease before conventional structural or functional deficits appear. Preliminary studies suggest that reduced vessel density may be identifiable in preperimetric glaucoma and glaucoma suspects, potentially serving as an early biomarker for disease. Additionally, OCTA parameters have shown correlations with visual field sensitivity, suggesting potential functional relevance of these vascular measurements. While challenges remain, including the need for standardized acquisition protocols, improved image quality metrics, and longitudinal data on progression, OCTA represents a significant addition to the diagnostic armamentarium with particular promise for detecting early vascular changes that may precede or contribute to glaucomatous damage.

Enhanced Depth Imaging and Swept-Source OCT

Advances in OCT technology have significantly improved imaging of deeper ocular structures relevant to glaucoma, particularly the lamina cribrosa and choroid. Enhanced depth imaging OCT (EDI-OCT) and swept-source OCT (SS-OCT) overcome the depth limitations of conventional spectral-domain OCT, allowing detailed visualization of these previously inaccessible structures. The lamina cribrosa, a key site of glaucomatous injury, can now be assessed for various parameters including thickness, curvature, depth, and focal defects. Studies have identified associations between laminar parameters and both glaucoma presence and severity. Particularly noteworthy is the potential prognostic value of laminar imaging, with some evidence suggesting that certain features, such as focal laminar defects, may predict localized RNFL progression and visual field deterioration. Similarly, improved choroidal imaging has revealed associations between choroidal thickness and various forms of glaucoma, though the clinical significance and utility of these findings remain subjects of ongoing investigation. As normative databases expand and analysis algorithms improve, these deeper structural assessments may provide additional biomarkers for early diagnosis and risk stratification.

Functional Testing Innovations

Objective Perimetry

Traditional perimetry relies on subjective patient responses, introducing variability and requiring patient cooperation and reliability. Several emerging technologies aim to provide objective assessment of visual function, potentially offering earlier and more reliable detection of functional deficits. Multifocal visual evoked potential (mfVEP) technology measures cortical responses to visual stimuli, providing an objective assessment of the visual field. By recording electrical potentials from electrodes placed on the scalp, mfVEP can detect functional deficits without requiring subjective patient responses. Studies have demonstrated that mfVEP can detect visual field abnormalities in patients with normal standard automated perimetry, suggesting potential for earlier diagnosis. However, technical complexity, lengthy testing time, and significant inter-individual variability have limited widespread clinical adoption. Multifocal electroretinography (mfERG) provides objective assessment of retinal ganglion cell function. By measuring electrical responses from discrete retinal regions, mfERG can identify localized functional deficits. Adaptations specifically designed for glaucoma assessment, including photopic negative response evaluation, show promise for detecting early functional changes.

Portable and Home-Based Visual Field Testing

The development of tablet-based and smartphone-based perimetry applications represents another significant innovation aimed at increasing accessibility and frequency of visual field assessment. These technologies enable testing outside traditional clinical settings, potentially allowing more frequent monitoring and earlier detection of progression. Tablet-based suprathreshold testing strategies have demonstrated reasonable concordance with conventional automated perimetry. The Melbourne rapid fields test, for example, has shown 95% agreement with Humphrey visual fields for detection of glaucomatous defects. Similarly, smartphone-based applications such as Visual Fields Easy have demonstrated promise for screening and monitoring purposes. Virtual reality-based perimetry, incorporating head-mounted displays, offers potential advantages including standardized testing environment, control over background illumination, and real-time eye tracking. Early comparison studies have shown promising correlations with conventional perimetry results. While these portable technologies do not yet match the precision of standard clinical perimeters, they offer substantial potential for increased testing frequency, home monitoring, telehealth integration, and expanded access in resource-limited settings.

Artificial Intelligence and Machine Learning

Perhaps the most transformative force in glaucoma diagnostics is the application of artificial intelligence (AI) and machine learning. These computational approaches can identify patterns and relationships in complex datasets that may not be apparent to human observers, potentially revolutionizing how we detect and monitor glaucoma.

Deep learning systems have demonstrated remarkable capability in analyzing ophthalmic images for glaucoma detection. Convolutional neural networks trained on thousands of fundus photographs and OCT images can distinguish glaucomatous from normal eyes with sensitivity and specificity comparable to or exceeding expert clinicians. A pioneering study (54) demonstrated a deep learning system capable of detecting referable glaucomatous optic neuropathy from fundus photographs with an area under the curve of 0.942, sensitivity of 96.4%, and specificity of 87.2%. Beyond simple classification, AI algorithms can now identify specific features associated with glaucoma, segment ocular structures, and quantify parameters relevant to diagnosis. These capabilities are increasingly being incorporated into commercial imaging platforms, enhancing clinical workflow and standardizing assessment.

AI approaches excel at integrating diverse data types to detect subtle progression patterns and predict future disease trajectory. Machine learning algorithms can incorporate structural imaging, functional testing, clinical risk factors, and demographic information to generate personalized risk assessments and progression predictions. It was demonstrated that machine learning algorithms integrating functional, structural, and demographic data could predict future visual field damage with significantly greater accuracy than conventional methods or human experts. These predictive models offer potential for identifying high-risk patients who may benefit from earlier or more aggressive intervention. The integration of large-scale electronic health record data with advanced analytics promises to generate insights that controlled clinical trials cannot provide. By analyzing patterns across millions of patient encounters, AI systems can identify novel risk factors, treatment response predictors, and disease subgroups. The IRIS® Registry (Intelligent Research in Sight), the American Academy of Ophthalmology's clinical data registry, contains data from over 60 million unique patients and has enabled large-scale analyses of glaucoma practice patterns, treatment outcomes, and disease progression. As these datasets grow and analytical methods improve, they will increasingly inform personalized clinical decision-making.

Intraocular Pressure Fluctuation and Continuous Monitoring

Recognition of IOP fluctuation as an independent risk factor for glaucoma progression has driven development of continuous monitoring technologies. The Triggerfish®

contact lens sensor (Sensimed AG) measures changes in corneal curvature as a surrogate for IOP fluctuations, providing 24-hour profiles of relative pressure patterns. While not providing absolute IOP values, these continuous measurements reveal nocturnal patterns and fluctuations that may have significant clinical relevance. Implantable IOP sensors represent the next frontier, with devices such as the Eyemate® system (Implandata Ophthalmic Products GmbH) demonstrating capability for long-term continuous monitoring. As these technologies mature and miniaturize, they may fundamentally change how we conceptualize IOP assessment and management.

Molecular and Genetic Biomarkers

Advances in proteomics, metabolomics, and genomics are identifying molecular signatures associated with glaucoma development, progression, and treatment response. Analysis of aqueous humor, tears, blood, and even imaging-derived radiomic features may yield biomarkers for early detection, disease subtyping, and personalized therapy selection. While most molecular biomarkers remain investigational, several gene variants associated with glaucoma risk (including MYOC, OPTN, TBK1, and CDKN2B-AS1) have transitioned into clinical testing. As our understanding of genetic contributions to glaucoma grows, expanded genetic testing may enable more precise risk stratification and potentially genotype-directed therapies.

Figure 7.1 provides an illustration of the comparison between OCT imaging to AI-assisted diagnostics, as explained in the previous text. To summarize, the

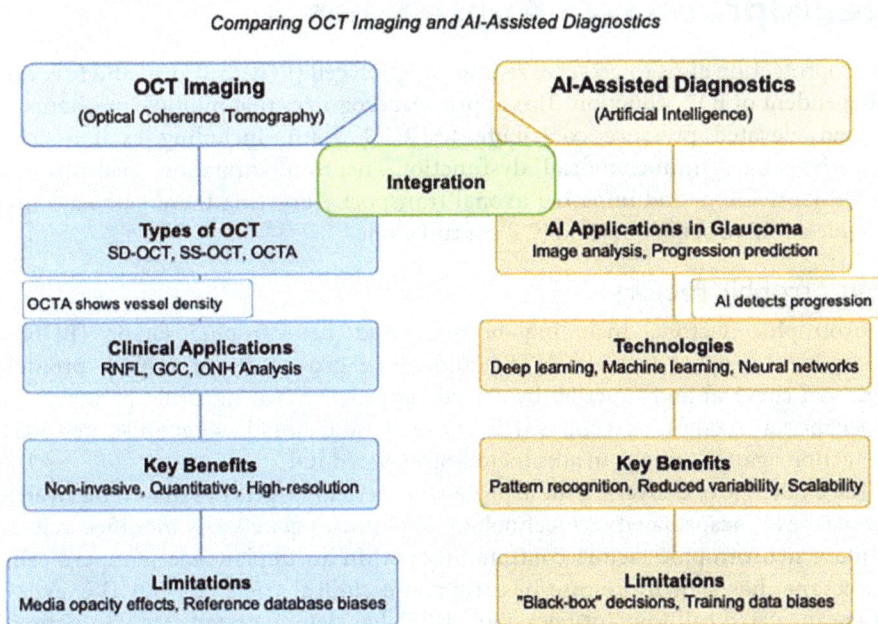

Figure 7.1 Comparison of OCT imaging and AI-assistant diagnostics.

diagnostic landscape for glaucoma is undergoing a remarkable transformation driven by technological innovation, computational advances, and deepening biological understanding. These emerging tools promise earlier detection, more precise characterization, and more sensitive progression monitoring than conventional approaches. While most remain in research or early clinical implementation stages, their continued development and validation will likely enable a paradigm shift from reactive disease management to proactive, preventive care based on comprehensive risk assessment and earliest possible intervention.

SECTION 2—EXPERIMENTAL THERAPIES AND STEM CELL RESEARCH

While intraocular pressure reduction remains the mainstay of current glaucoma management, the irreversible nature of glaucomatous damage and the recognition that many patients continue to progress despite well-controlled IOP have intensified the search for novel therapeutic approaches. The ultimate goals of protecting remaining neurons (neuroprotection), restoring lost neuronal function (neurorestoration), and regenerating damaged neural tissue (neuroregeneration) represent the new frontiers in glaucoma treatment. This section explores emerging experimental therapies that target these ambitious objectives, with particular emphasis on neuroprotective strategies, gene therapy, stem cell applications, and novel drug delivery systems.

Neuroprotective Approaches

Neuroprotection aims to preserve retinal ganglion cell (RGC) survival and function independent of IOP reduction. This approach recognizes that multiple mechanisms beyond elevated pressure contribute to RGC death, including excitotoxicity, oxidative stress, mitochondrial dysfunction, neuroinflammation, neurotrophic factor deprivation, and impaired axonal transport. Targeting these pathways may provide additive benefit beyond IOP control alone.

Neurotrophic Factors

Neurotrophic factors, including brain-derived neurotrophic factor (BDNF), ciliary neurotrophic factor (CNTF), and nerve growth factor (NGF), promote neuronal survival and function by activating pro-survival signaling pathways. In experimental models, exogenous delivery of these factors has demonstrated RGC protection against various insults including elevated IOP.

The challenge of delivering these proteins to retinal targets has driven innovative approaches. Encapsulated cell technology, which uses genetically modified cells to produce neurotrophic factors continuously within an implantable semipermeable membrane, has shown promise in early-phase clinical trials. NT-501 (Renexus®), an encapsulated cell implant releasing CNTF, has demonstrated safety in patients with retinitis pigmentosa and macular telangiectasia, providing proof-of-concept for potential glaucoma applications.

Gene therapy approaches, discussed in more detail later, offer another strategy for sustained local production of neurotrophic factors. Viral vector-mediated expression of BDNF or CNTF has demonstrated RGC protection in various animal models of optic nerve injury and glaucoma. These approaches seek to overcome the short half-life and poor bioavailability that have limited conventional protein delivery methods.

Targeting Excitotoxicity and Oxidative Stress

Excitotoxicity, predominantly mediated by excessive glutamate signaling, represents a key mechanism of RGC damage in glaucoma. Memantine, an NMDA receptor antagonist used in Alzheimer's disease, has been extensively studied for glaucoma neuroprotection. Despite promising results in animal models, phase 3 clinical trials in glaucoma patients failed to demonstrate significant benefit, highlighting the challenges of translating neuroprotective strategies to clinical practice.

Antioxidant approaches target the oxidative damage implicated in RGC death. While numerous antioxidant compounds have shown protection in preclinical models, clinical translation has proven challenging. Novel approaches include mitochondria-targeted antioxidants such as MitoQ, which concentrate within mitochondria to counteract oxidative damage at its primary source, and activation of endogenous antioxidant pathways through Nrf2 agonists like sulforaphane.

Anti-Inflammatory and Immunomodulatory Strategies

Neuroinflammation, characterized by microglial activation and increased pro-inflammatory cytokines, contributes to RGC damage in glaucoma. Anti-inflammatory approaches ranging from broad-spectrum agents like minocycline to targeted inhibitors of specific inflammatory mediators have demonstrated varying degrees of neuroprotection in experimental models.

The recognition of autoimmune components in glaucomatous damage, where the immune system may inappropriately target retinal antigens, has prompted investigation of immunomodulatory approaches. T cell-directed therapies and vaccination strategies aimed at inducing protective immunity have shown promise in animal models but remain in early experimental stages for human application.

Gene Therapy Approaches

Gene therapy offers the potential for sustained therapeutic effects through targeted genetic modification of ocular tissues. The eye represents an ideal target for gene therapy due to its accessibility, immune privilege, and small tissue volume requiring treatment. Several approaches are under investigation for glaucoma:

IOP-Lowering Gene Therapy
Gene therapy strategies targeting aqueous humor dynamics aim to provide sustained IOP reduction through a single intervention. Approaches include

viral vector-mediated expression of prostaglandin pathway enzymes to enhance uveoscleral outflow, modulation of the conventional outflow pathway through trabecular meshwork-targeted gene delivery, and reduction of aqueous production through ciliary epithelium-directed therapy. A phase 1 clinical trial of ADVM-022, an adeno-associated virus (AAV) vector expressing aflibercept for neovascular AMD, has demonstrated sustained therapeutic protein expression following a single intravitreal injection, providing proof-of-concept for similar approaches in glaucoma. Early-stage clinical trials of gene therapy specifically for IOP reduction are now underway, including TGR-1801, which uses an AAV vector to express a prostaglandin analog in the anterior segment.

Neuroprotective Gene Therapy

Gene therapy offers an elegant solution to the challenge of delivering neuroprotective proteins to retinal targets. By introducing genes encoding neurotrophic factors, anti-apoptotic proteins, or antioxidant enzymes directly into RGCs or supporting cells, sustained local production can be achieved without repeated interventions. A pioneering study (55) demonstrated that a single intravitreal injection of an AAV vector expressing BDNF provided significant RGC protection in a primate model of optic nerve transection, with effects persisting throughout the five-month study period. Similar approaches using CNTF, GDNF, and other neuroprotective factors have shown promise in various animal models of glaucoma and optic neuropathy. Beyond neurotrophic factors, gene therapy can target specific pathways implicated in RGC death. For example, viral vector-mediated expression of anti-apoptotic proteins like Bcl-2 or inhibitors of critical cell death pathways offers potential for interrupting the final common pathway of RGC loss. Similarly, expression of superoxide dismutase or other antioxidant enzymes could provide sustained protection against oxidative damage.

Stem Cell Approaches

Stem cell-based strategies represent perhaps the most ambitious frontier in glaucoma therapeutics, with the ultimate goal of replacing lost RGCs and restoring visual function. While formidable challenges remain, significant progress has occurred in several key areas.

The successful generation of RGCs from various stem cell sources, including embryonic stem cells (ESCs), induced pluripotent stem cells (iPSCs), and Müller glia-derived stem cells, has been a critical first step. Protocols now exist for differentiating these stem cells into RGCs with appropriate morphological and electrophysiological characteristics, expressing typical RGC markers like RBPMS, Brn3a, and Thy–1.

The next major hurdle involves successful integration of transplanted RGCs into existing retinal circuitry. It was demonstrated that transplanted mouse ESC-derived RGCs could migrate into the ganglion cell layer, extend axons, and form synaptic connections in mice with damaged retinas (56). However, the efficiency of integration and functional recovery remain limited, with most transplanted cells failing to establish appropriate connections.

Perhaps the greatest challenge is axonal pathfinding and regeneration. Transplanted RGCs must extend axons through the optic nerve head, navigate the optic chiasm, and form appropriate connections in central visual targets. Various approaches to overcome inhibitory signals and promote axon growth are under investigation, including manipulation of cell-intrinsic growth programs, neutralization of extrinsic inhibitory factors, and creation of permissive growth environments through biomaterial scaffolds.

A more immediately feasible application of stem cell technology may be neuroprotection rather than cell replacement. Transplanted stem cells, even without full integration, can secrete neurotrophic factors, modulate inflammation, and provide structural support that enhances survival of remaining RGCs. Mesenchymal stem cells (MSCs) have demonstrated particular promise in this regard. Intravitreal injection of MSCs has shown neuroprotective effects in various animal models of glaucoma and optic nerve injury, predominantly through paracrine mechanisms rather than direct cell replacement. Clinical trials of MSC therapy for glaucoma and other optic neuropathies are currently underway, with early results suggesting favorable safety profiles and potential efficacy signals that warrant further investigation.

Retinal Organoids and Disease Modeling

Stem cell-derived retinal organoids—three-dimensional structures that recapitulate key aspects of retinal development and organization—offer unprecedented opportunities for disease modeling and drug screening. Patient-derived iPSCs can be differentiated into retinal organoids that reproduce disease phenotypes, enabling mechanistic studies and therapeutic testing in a human cellular context. For glaucoma, organoids developed from patients with specific genetic forms of the disease allow investigation of pathological mechanisms and potential interventions in a controlled system. Additionally, these organoids provide platforms for high-throughput screening of neuroprotective compounds, potentially accelerating drug discovery for glaucoma.

Novel Drug Delivery Systems

The challenge of achieving sustained therapeutic concentrations at target tissues while minimizing side effects has driven significant innovation in ocular drug delivery. Several emerging approaches hold particular promise for glaucoma therapeutics: Various implantable devices for sustained medication release are under development for glaucoma. These range from biodegradable intracameral implants that release prostaglandin analogs over several months to reservoir-based systems capable of delivering multiple medications with programmable release profiles. The Bimatoprost SR implant (Durysta™), approved in 2020, represents the first FDA-approved sustained-release implant for glaucoma, providing IOP reduction for four to six months following a single intracameral injection. Next-generation implants aim to extend duration further and incorporate novel neuroprotective agents alongside IOP-lowering medications.

Nanoparticle formulations offer potential for enhanced drug penetration, targeted delivery, and sustained release. Polymeric nanoparticles, liposomes, dendrimers, and other nanoscale carriers can encapsulate conventional glaucoma medications or novel therapeutic agents, potentially improving efficacy while reducing dosing frequency and side effects.

For gene therapy and nucleic acid-based therapeutics like siRNA, nanoparticles may provide non-viral alternatives to viral vectors, potentially offering improved safety profiles and larger genetic payload capacity. Similarly, nanoparticle systems may enable more efficient delivery of neuroprotective proteins, overcoming the bioavailability limitations that have hampered conventional protein delivery approaches.

To conclude, the experimental therapies discussed in this section represent ambitious attempts to move beyond IOP reduction toward direct protection, restoration, and regeneration of neural tissues affected by glaucoma. While many remain in preclinical or early clinical stages, they collectively offer hope for transformative advances in glaucoma management. The continued evolution of these approaches, coupled with improved understanding of glaucoma pathophysiology and enhanced methods for patient-specific phenotyping, promises a future where treatment can be tailored to specific disease mechanisms and stages, potentially preventing blindness even in cases refractory to current therapies.

SECTION 3—FUTURE DIRECTIONS IN GLAUCOMA CARE

The landscape of glaucoma management is poised for transformation through the convergence of technological innovation, data science, personalized medicine, and evolving healthcare delivery models. While current approaches have significantly reduced blindness from glaucoma, substantial challenges remain, including delayed diagnosis, suboptimal treatment adherence, and continued progression despite intervention in many patients. This section explores emerging paradigms that promise to address these challenges and fundamentally alter how glaucoma is detected, monitored, and treated in the coming decades.

The concept of precision medicine—tailoring prevention and treatment strategies to individual characteristics, environment, and lifestyle—is gaining traction in glaucoma care. This approach recognizes the heterogeneity of glaucoma and seeks to match interventions to specific disease mechanisms, risk factors, and patient characteristics.

Molecular Phenotyping and Biomarker-Guided Therapy

Advances in genomics, proteomics, and metabolomics are yielding insights into molecular mechanisms underlying different glaucoma subtypes. These technologies enable more precise disease characterization beyond traditional clinical parameters. For example, aqueous humor proteomics has identified distinct protein expression patterns in different glaucoma types, potentially allowing targeted interventions based on specific pathological processes. Genome-wide association studies have identified numerous genetic variants associated with glaucoma risk and progression. As our understanding of these genetic factors deepens, genetic testing may inform individualized risk assessment and potentially guide therapy selection. A landmark study (57), analyzing genetic data from over 140,000 participants, identified 133 genetic variants associated with IOP and primary open-angle glaucoma, demonstrating the complex genetic architecture of these traits and laying groundwork for future genetic risk stratification. The integration of multiple data types—genetic, molecular, structural, functional, and clinical—promises more comprehensive patient profiling and personalized treatment selection. Machine learning approaches are increasingly being applied to identify patterns within these complex datasets, potentially revealing novel disease subtypes and prediction models that could inform individualized management strategies.

Pharmacogenomics and Treatment Response Prediction

Pharmacogenomic approaches aim to predict individual responses to medications based on genetic factors, potentially enabling therapy selection that maximizes efficacy while minimizing side effects. While in early stages for glaucoma, studies have identified genetic variants associated with differential responses to various medication classes. Beyond genetics, integration of clinical, demographic, and structural/functional parameters may enhance prediction of treatment outcomes. Predictive models could guide initial therapy selection, potentially replacing the current step-wise approach with more targeted initial intervention. Such models might also identify patients likely to benefit from early surgical intervention versus those best managed with conservative approaches.

Telehealth and Remote Monitoring

The COVID-19 pandemic accelerated adoption of telehealth across medicine, including ophthalmology. For glaucoma, remote care models offer potential solutions to challenges of access, monitoring frequency, and continuity of care. Home-based IOP monitoring devices, ranging from rebound tonometers to contact lens sensors, enable more frequent pressure assessment outside the clinical setting. These measurements may reveal diurnal fluctuations and treatment response patterns not captured during office visits, potentially improving therapeutic decision-making. Similarly, home-based visual function testing using tablet computers, smartphones, or dedicated devices allows more frequent assessment of functional status. These technologies range from basic visual field screening to more sophisticated perimetry applications that correlate reasonably well with standard clinical tests. Home monitoring of medication adherence through smart bottles, electronic caps, or mobile applications provides insights into actual medication usage patterns, potentially enabling timely intervention for non-adherence. Integration of these diverse home monitoring data streams could create comprehensive remote assessment systems that supplement in-person evaluation.

Hybrid Care Models

Rather than replacing traditional care entirely, telehealth will likely become integrated into hybrid models combining remote and in-person elements. Such models might include remote monitoring with algorithm-guided triage determining the need and timing for in-person evaluation. This approach could increase effective monitoring frequency while optimizing utilization of clinical resources. Virtual visits might alternate with in-person assessments for stable patients, potentially increasing convenience and adherence to follow-up schedules. Artificial intelligence-based image analysis could enable remote review of optic nerve photographs or OCT scans obtained at satellite locations, extending specialist expertise to underserved areas.

Artificial Intelligence and Clinical Decision Support

Artificial intelligence (AI) applications in glaucoma extend beyond image analysis to comprehensive clinical decision support. These systems aim not to replace clinician judgment but to augment decision-making with data-driven insights.

AI algorithms integrating structural, functional, and clinical data can predict individualized disease trajectories with potentially greater accuracy than traditional methods. These predictions could inform decisions regarding treatment escalation, target pressure selection, and follow-up intervals. A study (58) demonstrated that a deep learning system trained on visual fields and OCT data could forecast future field changes more accurately than existing clinical prediction tools. Such forecasting capabilities may eventually enable truly preventive intervention, targeting patients at highest risk for progression before significant damage occurs.

AI-based systems may eventually recommend personalized treatment regimens based on multiple patient factors and expected outcomes. These recommendations could incorporate considerations of efficacy, side effects, adherence probability, cost, and patient preferences, potentially optimizing the complex balance of factors that influence treatment success.

For surgical intervention, AI could assist in procedure selection and timing based on individual risk profiles and surgical outcome predictions. As surgical options continue to diversify, such decision support may become increasingly valuable for navigating complex treatment algorithms.

Beyond technological advances, innovations in healthcare delivery models and policy will significantly impact future glaucoma care. Population-based screening using low-cost technologies and risk stratification algorithms may enable earlier detection in high-risk communities. Targeted screening approaches based on demographic, genetic, and clinical risk factors could improve cost-effectiveness compared to universal screening. Risk-stratified care models, where follow-up intensity and treatment approach are calibrated to individual risk profiles, may optimize resource allocation while maintaining or improving outcomes. Such models require robust risk prediction tools but could significantly enhance healthcare system efficiency.

Value-Based Care Models

As healthcare systems increasingly emphasize value rather than volume, glaucoma care delivery will likely evolve toward outcomes-based approaches. These models incentivize preservation of visual function rather than simply providing services, potentially encouraging more effective preventive care and earlier intervention. Cost-effectiveness will play an increasingly important role in technology adoption and treatment selection. Comparative effectiveness research examining not only clinical outcomes but also economic impacts and quality of life effects will guide implementation of new approaches within resource-constrained systems.

The future directions described previously present not only opportunities but also significant challenges and ethical considerations. Issues of data privacy, algorithm transparency, healthcare disparities, and equitable access to advanced technologies must be addressed to ensure that innovations benefit all patients.

The digital divide remains a significant concern, with potential for technological advances to exacerbate rather than reduce healthcare disparities if not implemented thoughtfully. Ensuring that underserved populations benefit from innovations in glaucoma care will require deliberate policy efforts and technology development focused on accessibility and affordability.

Additionally, the integration of AI into clinical decision-making raises questions about responsibility, liability, and the appropriate balance between algorithmic recommendation and clinician judgment. Developing clear frameworks for these issues will be essential as AI applications become more pervasive in glaucoma management.

Figure 7.2 provides a schematic illustration of future directions in glaucoma therapies.

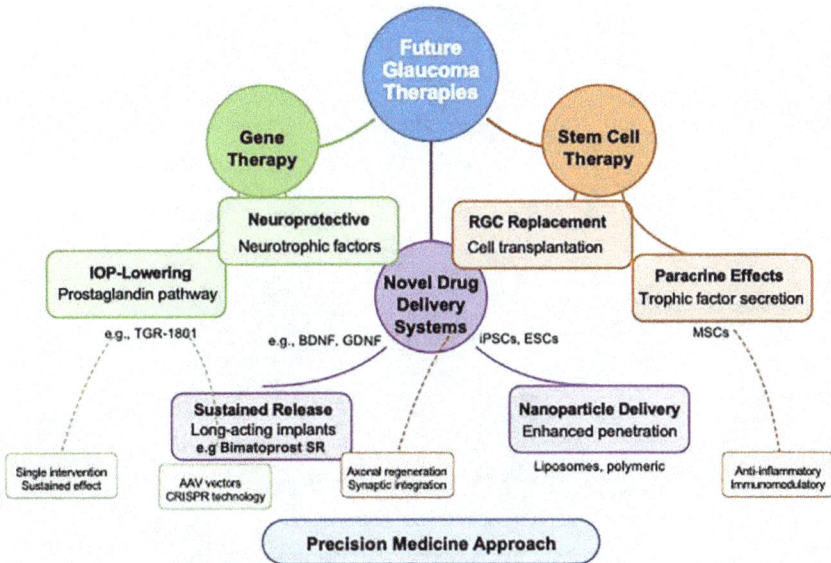

Figure 7.2 Future directions in glaucoma therapies.

In conclusion, the future of glaucoma care will likely be characterized by more personalized, proactive, and patient-centered approaches enabled by technological innovation and evolving healthcare models. Integration of precision medicine, telehealth, artificial intelligence, and novel delivery systems promises to address current limitations in diagnosis, monitoring, and treatment. While significant challenges remain in development, validation, implementation, and access, these emerging paradigms collectively offer the potential for substantial improvements in outcomes for individuals with or at risk for glaucoma.

CHAPTER 8
SPECIAL CONSIDERATIONS IN GLAUCOMA MANAGEMENT

While previous chapters have addressed the fundamental principles of glaucoma diagnosis and treatment, certain patient populations and clinical scenarios require modified approaches that extend beyond standard management protocols. The heterogeneity of glaucoma necessitates individualized care strategies that consider not only the specific disease mechanism but also patient characteristics, comorbidities, resources, and social context. This chapter examines several important scenarios that demand specialized knowledge and tailored management approaches.

Pediatric glaucoma presents unique challenges that distinguish it from adult disease. The developing eye responds differently to elevated intraocular pressure, with potential for globe enlargement and significant refractive changes. Examination often requires specialized techniques and anesthesia, while treatment must consider the long life expectancy of these young patients and the potential for amblyopia development. Surgical intervention frequently serves as primary therapy rather than the stepped approach typical in adult disease, creating distinct management considerations for this vulnerable population.

Secondary glaucomas encompass a diverse group of disorders where elevated intraocular pressure results from identifiable ocular or systemic conditions. These forms often demonstrate unique pathophysiology, natural history, and treatment responses compared to primary glaucomas. From pseudoexfoliation to pigmentary mechanisms, from inflammatory to neovascular processes, these conditions require targeted approaches addressing both the underlying cause and the resultant pressure elevation.

Systemic diseases significantly impact glaucoma management through multiple mechanisms. Certain systemic conditions directly influence glaucoma risk and progression, while others affect treatment options through medication interactions or contraindications. Moreover, balancing glaucoma care with management of serious systemic comorbidities creates prioritization challenges, particularly in patients with limited life expectancy or significant functional impairment from non-ocular conditions.

Finally, resource limitations—whether financial, geographic, or infrastructural—profoundly influence feasible management approaches in many settings. Developing cost-effective, sustainable care models represents a critical challenge for addressing glaucoma globally. Innovative approaches to screening, diagnosis, and treatment that maximize visual outcomes within significant resource constraints offer potential solutions for reducing global blindness from this disease.

DOI: 10.1201/9781003646693-8

By examining these special considerations in glaucoma management, this chapter provides a framework for adapting fundamental principles to the complex realities of diverse patient populations and practice environments. The ability to recognize these unique scenarios and modify standard approaches accordingly represents an essential skill for comprehensive glaucoma care.

SECTION I—GLAUCOMA IN PEDIATRIC POPULATIONS

Pediatric glaucoma represents a heterogeneous group of disorders that cause elevated intraocular pressure with potential for optic nerve damage and visual impairment in children. While considerably less common than adult glaucoma, childhood forms present unique diagnostic and management challenges due to examination difficulties, distinctive pathophysiology, different natural history, and significant long-term implications for visual development. This section examines the classification, diagnosis, and management of pediatric glaucoma, with emphasis on the specialized approaches required for this vulnerable population.

Pediatric glaucoma is broadly categorized as primary or secondary. Primary forms include primary congenital glaucoma (PCG), which is present from birth or early infancy, and juvenile open-angle glaucoma (JOAG), which typically manifests between the ages of 4 and 35 years. Secondary forms arise from various conditions including anterior segment dysgenesis (e.g., Axenfeld–Rieger syndrome, Peters anomaly), aphakia/pseudophakia, uveitis, trauma, steroid use, and associated systemic disorders (e.g., Sturge-Weber syndrome, neurofibromatosis).

Primary congenital glaucoma, the most common form of pediatric glaucoma, demonstrates significant geographical and ethnic variation in incidence. In Western populations, PCG occurs in approximately 1 in 10,000–20,000 live births, while higher rates are reported in regions with greater consanguinity. The condition predominantly results from abnormal development of the anterior chamber angle and trabecular meshwork (trabeculodysgenesis), leading to impaired aqueous outflow.

Juvenile open-angle glaucoma, though clinically similar to adult-onset POAG, typically demonstrates more aggressive progression and often stronger genetic associations. Mutations in the MYOC gene, encoding myocilin, account for 8–36% of JOAG cases, with autosomal dominant inheritance and high penetrance.

The clinical manifestations of pediatric glaucoma vary considerably with age of onset and underlying mechanism. In infants with congenital glaucoma, the classic triad of epiphora (excessive tearing), photophobia (light sensitivity), and blepharospasm (eyelid squeezing) results from corneal epithelial edema secondary to elevated IOP. Physical findings may include corneal enlargement and haziness, Haab striae (horizontal breaks in Descemet's membrane), increased corneal diameter (>12 mm before 1 year of age), and buphthalmos (globe enlargement).

In older children, symptoms may more closely resemble adult glaucoma, though myopia development or progression due to axial length elongation may represent the earliest sign. However, children rarely complain of visual loss, and subtle central vision decline may be difficult to detect, making regular screening and comprehensive examination essential.

The diagnosis of pediatric glaucoma presents significant challenges. Examination often requires sedation or general anesthesia, particularly in infants and young children. Under anesthesia, essential measurements include intraocular pressure (recognizing that anesthetic agents influence IOP), corneal diameter, axial length, and comprehensive assessment of the anterior segment and optic nerve. The Childhood Glaucoma Research Network (CGRN) has established consensus examination guidelines and diagnostic criteria for various forms of childhood glaucoma to standardize evaluation and reporting.

Intraocular pressure measurement requires specialized approaches in children. While Goldmann applanation tonometry remains the gold standard for cooperative patients, alternatives such as rebound tonometry (iCare), pneumatonometry, Tono-Pen, and hand-held applanation devices provide valuable options for younger or less cooperative children. Interpretation must consider normal age-adjusted ranges and the effect of examination conditions. Gonioscopy plays a crucial role in identifying angle abnormalities characteristic of various pediatric glaucoma types. In primary congenital glaucoma, the angle typically demonstrates an immature appearance with anterior insertion of the iris, obscured or poorly developed angle structures, and excessive iris processes or sheet-like tissue overlying the trabecular meshwork. Direct visualization of these features aids in differential diagnosis and surgical planning.

Optic nerve and visual field assessment presents particular difficulties in children but remains essential for diagnosis and monitoring. Fundus photography, when feasible, provides valuable documentation of optic nerve appearance. Quantitative imaging with optical coherence tomography is increasingly employed, with pediatric normative databases now available for many devices. Visual field testing, though challenging in young children, becomes increasingly feasible and reliable after ages 7–8, with modified testing strategies and careful encouragement.

The management paradigm for pediatric glaucoma differs fundamentally from adult disease, with surgery typically serving as primary therapy rather than a later intervention after medication failure. This approach reflects both the pathophysiology of many pediatric forms (particularly those involving structural abnormalities of the outflow pathways) and concerns regarding long-term medication adherence, side effects, and efficacy in the developing eye.

Angle surgery represents the initial intervention for primary congenital glaucoma, directly addressing the underlying trabeculodysgenesis. Goniotomy, performed under direct visualization through a clear cornea, creates incisions in the abnormal trabecular tissue to establish aqueous communication with Schlemm's canal. Trabeculotomy ab externo, which opens the canal from the outside, serves as an alternative when corneal cloudiness precludes adequate visualization for goniotomy. A landmark study (59) demonstrated success rates of 80–90% with initial angle surgery for primary congenital glaucoma diagnosed before one year of age, with lower success rates in later-onset cases or those with associated ocular anomalies. Combined trabeculotomy-trabeculectomy, circumferential 360-degree trabeculotomy using illuminated microcatheters, and other modifications may offer advantages for selected cases.

When angle surgery fails, filtering procedures including trabeculectomy with antimetabolites or glaucoma drainage device implantation become necessary. These interventions demonstrate higher complication rates in children compared to adults, with increased risk of hypotony, choroidal effusion, tube-related complications, and bleb-related infections. Cyclodestructive procedures typically represent a last resort when other interventions have failed.

For juvenile open-angle glaucoma, the surgical approach more closely resembles adult management, though earlier intervention may be warranted given the aggressive natural history. Newer micro-invasive glaucoma surgeries have limited evidence in pediatric populations but may eventually offer additional options with favorable risk profiles.

While surgery represents primary therapy for most congenital and infantile glaucomas, medical management plays important roles in specific scenarios: as temporizing treatment before surgery, as adjunctive therapy following partially successful surgical intervention, as primary treatment for certain secondary glaucomas (e.g., uveitic, steroid-induced), and for most cases of juvenile open-angle glaucoma.

Prostaglandin analogs, beta-blockers, alpha-2 agonists, and carbonic anhydrase inhibitors are all employed in pediatric glaucoma, though important considerations distinguish their use from adult practice. Prostaglandin analogs demonstrate variable efficacy in children, particularly those with congenital glaucoma. Beta-blockers warrant particular caution in infants due to potential systemic effects including bradycardia, bronchospasm, and hypoglycemia. Alpha-2 agonists are contraindicated in very young children and infants due to risk of central nervous system depression. Carbonic anhydrase inhibitors, both topical and oral, generally show good efficacy and acceptable safety, though long-term growth effects require monitoring.

The practical challenges of administering eye drops to infants and children cannot be overstated. Successful instillation often requires two caregivers, and adherence to multi-drug regimens poses substantial burdens on families. These factors further emphasize the preference for definitive surgical intervention when appropriate.

Beyond controlling intraocular pressure, comprehensive management of pediatric glaucoma must address several unique considerations:

- *Refractive correction* is essential, as these children often develop significant myopia, astigmatism, or anisometropia that requires optical correction to prevent amblyopia. Frequent refractive assessment is necessary given the potential for rapid changes during growth and following pressure-lowering interventions.
- *Amblyopia treatment*, including patching or atropine penalization of the better-seeing eye, represents a critical component of visual rehabilitation. The presence of glaucoma does not preclude aggressive amblyopia management, though coordination with glaucoma therapy is essential.
- *Developmental assessment and early intervention services* should be considered for children with significant visual impairment, as visual disability may impact motor, social, and cognitive development. Multidisciplinary care involving pediatric ophthalmologists, glaucoma specialists, optometrists, educators, and developmental specialists optimizes outcomes for affected children.
- *Long-term monitoring* extends throughout childhood and into adulthood, with lifetime risk of vision loss necessitating vigilant follow-up. As children mature, transition of care from pediatric to adult glaucoma specialists requires careful coordination to maintain continuity and treatment adherence.

Table 8.1 Differences between Adult and Pediatric Glaucoma

Feature	Adult Glaucoma	Pediatric Glaucoma
Onset	Usually after 40 years	Congenital or juvenile onset
IOP Presentation	Gradual elevation	Often dramatically elevated
Symptoms	Mostly asymptomatic	Photophobia, tearing, corneal enlargement
Management	Medications first	Surgery often first line
Prognosis	Variable	Often poorer without early treatment

Table 8.1 contrasts the clinical features of glaucoma in adults and pediatric populations. By emphasizing key differences in disease presentation, management approaches, and prognosis, this table underscores the importance of age-specific considerations in glaucoma care.

In summary, pediatric glaucoma presents distinct challenges that require specialized expertise in diagnosis, surgical technique, medical management, and developmental considerations. The stakes are particularly high given the potential for lifelong visual disability and associated developmental impacts if the condition is inadequately controlled. Early diagnosis, prompt surgical intervention for appropriate cases, comprehensive attention to visual rehabilitation, and continuity of care throughout development comprise the essential elements of effective management for this complex condition.

SECTION 2—MANAGING SECONDARY GLAUCOMAS

Secondary glaucomas encompass a diverse group of disorders in which elevated intraocular pressure and subsequent optic neuropathy result from identifiable ocular or systemic conditions. Unlike primary glaucomas, these forms have distinct underlying pathophysiologic mechanisms that often require specific therapeutic approaches targeting both the causative condition and the resultant pressure elevation. This section explores the management principles for several important categories of secondary glaucoma, highlighting the specialized considerations that distinguish their treatment from standard glaucoma protocols.

Lens-Related Glaucomas

Lens-related mechanisms represent common causes of secondary glaucoma, encompassing phacomorphic, phacolytic, lens particle, and pseudoexfoliation glaucomas.

Phacomorphic glaucoma results from angle closure induced by an advanced cataractous lens with increased thickness pushing the iris forward. Management primarily involves lens extraction, typically through small-incision phacoemulsification when possible. Medical therapy with topical aqueous suppressants, hyperosmotic agents, and occasionally oral acetazolamide serves to temporarily reduce pressure before surgery. Laser peripheral iridotomy may provide temporary relief by equalizing pressure between the anterior and posterior chambers but does not address the fundamental lens-related mechanism. Clear corneal approaches are generally preferred over scleral tunnel incisions, particularly in eyes with shallow anterior chambers. Careful attention to wound construction and size is essential to prevent postoperative wound leak and hypotony in these often crowded anterior segments.

Phacolytic glaucoma occurs when liquefied cortical material from a hypermature cataract leaks through an intact lens capsule, causing trabecular obstruction by macrophages engorged with lens protein. The condition typically presents with acute pressure elevation in an eye with longstanding mature cataract. While initial medical management resembles that for phacomorphic glaucoma, definitive treatment requires lens extraction. Surgical challenges include poor visualization due to cloudy cornea and aqueous, zonular weakness from lens maturity, and potential for intraoperative rupture of the fragile lens capsule. Thorough irrigation of residual lens material and viscoelastic is critical to prevent postoperative pressure spikes.

Pseudoexfoliation glaucoma, characterized by deposition of fibrillar material throughout anterior segment structures, presents distinct management challenges. These eyes demonstrate greater pressure fluctuation, higher peak pressures, and more rapid progression than primary open-angle glaucoma. Medical therapy follows similar principles to POAG but often requires earlier escalation to multiple medications. Laser trabeculoplasty demonstrates particularly good efficacy in pseudoexfoliation glaucoma, with studies showing success rates exceeding those observed in POAG. However, the effect may be less durable, requiring repeated treatment. Surgical intervention is frequently necessary, with special considerations including greater risk of zonular weakness during cataract surgery, reduced efficacy of trabecular micro-bypass procedures, and occasionally more favorable results with trabeculectomy compared to POAG. Long-term monitoring must account for the progressive nature of the underlying condition.

Inflammatory Glaucomas

Uveitic glaucoma presents complex management challenges requiring simultaneous control of inflammation and intraocular pressure. The mechanisms include trabecular meshwork obstruction by inflammatory cells and debris, trabeculitis with direct inflammatory damage to outflow structures, peripheral anterior synechiae formation, and steroid-induced pressure elevation.

Figure 8.1 shows a slit-lamp biomicroscopic image of a patient with herpetic uveitic glaucoma. Fine, pigmented keratic precipitates are visible on the corneal endothelium, together with inflammatory cells in the anterior chamber. Such findings are characteristic of viral anterior uveitis, a well-known cause of secondary glaucoma.

The cornerstone of management involves aggressive control of the underlying inflammation, typically with topical, periocular, or systemic corticosteroids depending on severity and etiology. Immunomodulatory therapy may be required for recalcitrant or recurrent inflammation. A landmark study (60) indicated that early introduction of immunomodulatory therapy in certain uveitic conditions

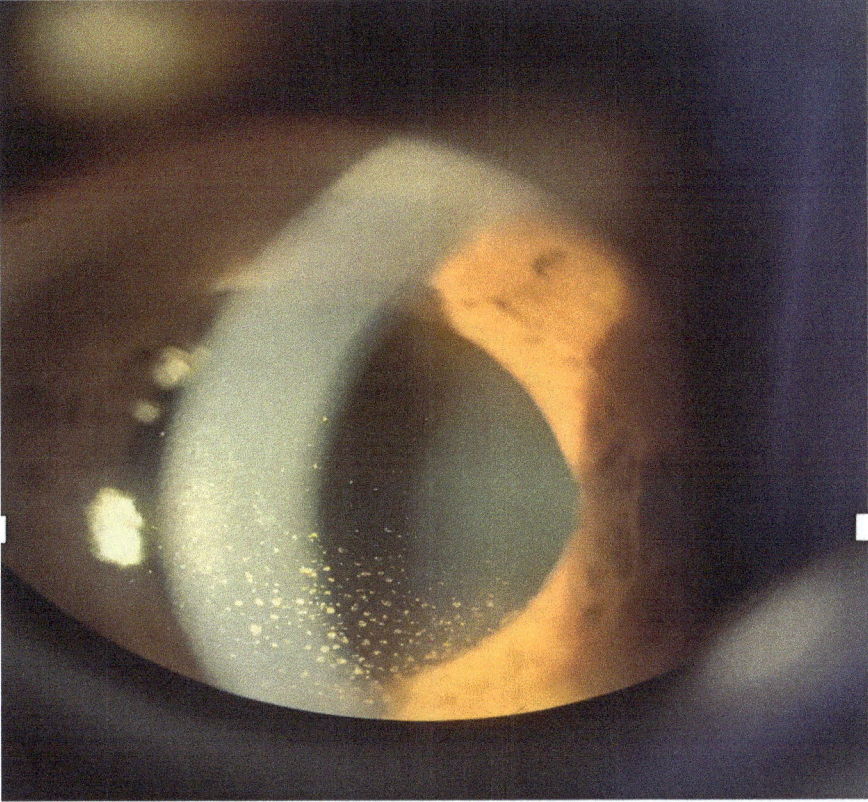

Figure 8.1 Herpetic uveitic glaucoma.

reduced the incidence of secondary glaucoma by approximately 50%, highlighting the importance of proactive inflammatory control.

Pressure management requires careful medication selection. Prostaglandin analogs warrant caution in active inflammatory disease due to potential exacerbation of inflammation and blood–ocular barrier disruption, though evidence for this concern remains equivocal. Beta-blockers, alpha-agonists, and carbonic anhydrase inhibitors generally represent safer options. Notably, oral acetazolamide may enhance the efficacy of immunosuppressive therapy in some inflammatory conditions, offering dual benefits. Surgical intervention often becomes necessary but carries higher complication rates than in primary glaucomas. Trabeculectomy demonstrates reduced success rates in uveitic eyes, with greater risk of hypotony and bleb failure. Antimetabolites are typically employed but require careful titration to balance antifibrotic effects against the risk of wound leak and hypotony. Glaucoma drainage devices show favorable outcomes in many uveitic cases, with some studies suggesting superior long-term success compared to trabeculectomy in these inflammatory conditions. However, tube occlusion by inflammatory debris and membrane formation around the plate remain unique complications requiring vigilant monitoring.

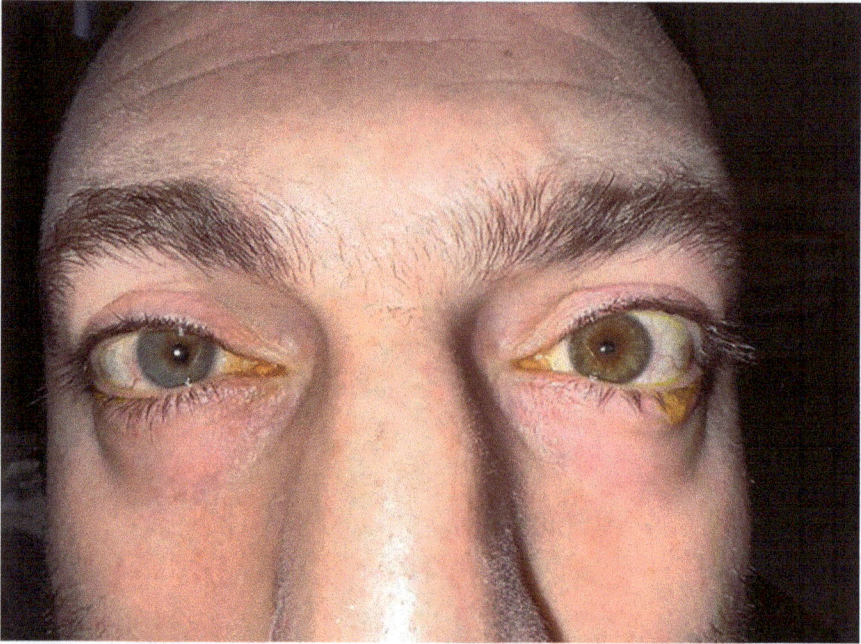

Figure 8.2 A male patient with Fuchs heterochromic iridocyclitis.

Figure 8.2 presents a clinical photograph of a 42-year-old male patient with Fuchs heterochromic iridocyclitis (FHI). The image illustrates the typical heterochromia of the iris caused by chronic low-grade inflammation, a condition that predisposes patients to secondary glaucoma due to trabecular meshwork dysfunction.

Neovascular Glaucoma

Neovascular glaucoma represents one of the most recalcitrant forms of secondary glaucoma, resulting from fibrovascular membrane formation over the angle structures in response to retinal ischemia. The predominant causes include proliferative diabetic retinopathy, central retinal vein occlusion, and ocular ischemic syndrome. Management principles emphasize early intervention for retinal ischemia to prevent neovascularization. Panretinal photocoagulation (PRP) remains the standard intervention for ablating ischemic retina and reducing angiogenic factors. In cases where media opacity precludes adequate laser delivery, transconjunctival cryotherapy provides an alternative approach.

Anti-vascular endothelial growth factor (anti-VEGF) agents have revo-lutionized early-stage management, causing rapid regression of iris and angle neovascularization. These agents serve dual purposes: preparing the eye for definitive PRP and transiently reducing intraocular pressure to create a window for additional interventions. While not a standalone cure, intravitreal bevacizumab or ranibizumab can convert an inflamed, congested eye with rubeosis into a more manageable condition amenable to definitive treatment.

Glaucoma drainage devices represent the preferred surgical approach when medical therapy fails to control pressure. The fibrovascular nature of the disease, with its propensity for hemorrhage and intense scarring, makes trabeculectomy less successful in these cases. Early tube ligation with staged activation may be necessary to prevent immediate postoperative hypotony in eyes with severely compromised outflow capacity. In end-stage, painful blind eyes, cyclodestructive procedures offer pressure control and comfort, though with minimal visual potential.

Traumatic Glaucoma

Traumatic glaucoma encompasses various mechanisms including angle recession, hyphema with trabecular obstruction, lens dislocation, and ghost cell glaucoma. Management strategies differ substantially based on the specific mechanism and timing. Acute management of hyphema-associated pressure elevation involves aqueous suppression with beta-blockers, alpha-agonists, and carbonic anhydrase inhibitors. Prostaglandin analogs are typically avoided due to their potential pro-inflammatory effects. Surgical evacuation becomes necessary for refractory pressure elevation, particularly with total hyphema or corneal blood staining. Antifibrinolytic agents like aminocaproic acid may reduce rebleed risk but can exacerbate clot formation and trabecular obstruction, warranting careful pressure monitoring during their use.

Angle recession glaucoma may develop months to years after blunt trauma. The management resembles that of primary open-angle glaucoma, though these cases often demonstrate more rapid progression and resistance to medical therapy. Surgical intervention frequently becomes necessary, with trabeculectomy, glaucoma drainage devices, or cyclophotocoagulation selected based on individual factors including age, corneal integrity, and prior surgical history.

Steroid-Induced Glaucoma

Steroid-induced ocular hypertension and glaucoma occur with all routes of corticosteroid administration, including topical, periocular, intravitreal, inhaled, and systemic delivery. The primary management approach involves steroid discontinuation or dose reduction when possible, with pressure typically normalizing within days to weeks after cessation, depending on the specific agent and duration of use. When continued steroid treatment is necessary for underlying disease control, switching to lower-potency steroids or non-steroidal alternatives may sufficiently reduce pressure in some cases. Fluorometholone, loteprednol, and rimexolone demonstrate reduced propensity for pressure elevation while retaining anti-inflammatory efficacy for milder conditions.

Medical glaucoma therapy follows standard approaches, with all major medication classes demonstrating efficacy. In refractory cases with ongoing steroid requirement, surgical intervention may become necessary, with options including trabeculectomy, glaucoma drainage devices, and minimally invasive procedures selected based on patient-specific factors and anticipated duration of steroid therapy.

In conclusion, the management of secondary glaucomas requires thorough understanding of the underlying pathophysiologic mechanisms coupled with targeted therapeutic approaches addressing both the causative condition and resultant pressure elevation. These diverse conditions often necessitate modification of standard glaucoma protocols, with greater emphasis on addressing the specific etiology while managing the consequent pressure-related optic neuropathy. Successful outcomes depend on prompt recognition of the underlying mechanism, early intervention to mitigate causative factors, and individualized treatment strategies that account for the unique characteristics of each secondary glaucoma subtype.

SECTION 3—GLAUCOMA AND SYSTEMIC DISEASES

The relationship between glaucoma and systemic disease is multidimensional and clinically significant. Systemic conditions can influence glaucoma risk, progression, diagnosis, and management through various mechanisms including direct effects on intraocular pressure, altered ocular blood flow, shared pathophysiological pathways, and treatment interactions. Understanding these complex relationships is essential for comprehensive glaucoma care, enabling clinicians to identify high-risk patients, optimize treatment approaches, and manage competing health priorities effectively. This section examines the interplay between glaucoma and several important systemic conditions, with emphasis on clinical implications for patient management.

Cardiovascular Diseases

The relationship between cardiovascular disease and glaucoma illustrates the complex interplay between systemic conditions and ocular health. Hypertension demonstrates a biphasic relationship with glaucoma risk and progression. Chronic hypertension may initially provide a protective effect by maintaining adequate optic nerve perfusion despite elevated intraocular pressure. However, long-standing hypertension ultimately promotes arteriosclerosis and endothelial dysfunction, compromising autoregulatory capacity and increasing susceptibility to pressure-induced damage. Management considerations include careful monitoring of both blood pressure and intraocular pressure, particularly in patients with advanced glaucoma. The common practice of administering antihypertensive medications at bedtime to reduce cardiovascular risk may inadvertently exacerbate nocturnal hypotension, potentially compromising optic nerve perfusion during sleep. In patients with progressive normal-tension glaucoma, 24-hour ambulatory blood pressure monitoring may reveal excessive nocturnal dips that contribute to disease progression. In such cases, collaboration with the patient's primary care physician or cardiologist to adjust the timing of antihypertensive medications can potentially improve ocular blood flow while maintaining systemic benefits. Conversely, systemic hypotension, whether primary or medication-induced, may adversely affect glaucoma by reducing ocular perfusion pressure. Studies have associated both low systolic blood pressure and large nocturnal blood pressure dips with increased glaucoma risk and progression, particularly in normal-tension glaucoma. The EMGT (Early Manifest Glaucoma Trial) demonstrated that lower systolic perfusion pressure was associated with increased glaucoma progression risk, with a hazard ratio of 1.42 for each 10 mmHg decrease. Consideration of ocular perfusion pressure—the difference between mean arterial pressure and intraocular pressure—is essential in patients with coexisting cardiovascular disease and glaucoma. Aggressive IOP lowering must be balanced against the risk of further compromising an already tenuous perfusion status, particularly in patients with autonomic dysfunction, advanced cardiovascular disease, or those on multiple antihypertensive medications.

Diabetes Mellitus

The relationship between diabetes and glaucoma remains somewhat controversial, with epidemiological studies showing inconsistent associations. However, several mechanisms potentially link these conditions, including microvascular damage, altered metabolism in the trabecular meshwork, and autonomic dysfunction affecting ocular blood flow regulation.

From a clinical management perspective, diabetic patients require special consideration in several aspects of glaucoma care. The selection of topical beta-blockers warrants caution due to their potential to mask symptoms of hypoglycemia and alter glucose metabolism. These effects are typically minimal with selective beta-blockers like betaxolol but may become significant with non-selective agents, particularly in patients with brittle diabetes or those on intensive insulin regimens.

Prostaglandin analogs generally represent safe options for diabetic patients, with limited systemic effects. However, these medications may exacerbate diabetic macular edema in susceptible individuals, necessitating regular macular assessment in patients with diabetic retinopathy who are using this drug class.

Steroid-induced pressure elevation occurs with greater frequency and severity in diabetic patients, requiring vigilant monitoring when corticosteroids are administered for diabetic macular edema or proliferative retinopathy. Alternative treatment approaches, including anti-VEGF therapy and non-steroidal options, may be preferable in patients with pre-existing glaucoma or ocular hypertension. Surgical considerations include increased risk of bleb failure following trabeculectomy in diabetic patients, potentially warranting more aggressive antimetabolite use or consideration of tube shunt procedures. Additionally, the increased susceptibility to infection requires meticulous postoperative care and prompt attention to potential bleb-related complications.

Obstructive Sleep Apnea

Emerging evidence links obstructive sleep apnea (OSA) with both increased glaucoma risk and progression. A meta-analysis (61) found that OSA was associated with a 1.65-fold increased risk of glaucoma, with stronger associations observed in studies using formal polysomnography for sleep apnea diagnosis. Multiple mechanisms potentially underlie this association, including repetitive hypoxic episodes leading to oxidative stress and inflammation, impaired optic nerve blood flow autoregulation, and direct effects of intracranial pressure fluctuations on the optic nerve. Clinically, patients with known OSA warrant regular comprehensive glaucoma assessment. Conversely, patients with normal-tension glaucoma and those demonstrating progression despite apparently well-controlled IOP should be evaluated for sleep apnea symptoms, with referral for polysomnography when appropriate. Continuous positive airway pressure (CPAP) therapy for OSA may stabilize glaucoma progression in some patients, though the potential for CPAP-associated IOP elevation requires monitoring, particularly in patients using the therapy for extended periods.

Thyroid Disorders

Thyroid eye disease presents unique challenges in glaucoma assessment and management. Elevated intraocular pressure may result from multiple mechanisms: increased episcleral venous pressure due to orbital congestion, mechanical compression of the globe by enlarged extraocular muscles, steroid-induced pressure elevation during inflammatory phase treatment, and restricted aqueous outflow from increased orbital pressure. Accurate tonometry proves challenging in these patients, as thickened extraocular muscles and increased orbital pressure can artifactually elevate IOP measurements, particularly with Goldmann applanation. Dynamic contour tonometry or rebound tonometry may provide more accurate assessment in such cases. Management requires collaboration between glaucoma specialists and oculoplastic surgeons, with orbital decompression sometimes necessary before definitive glaucoma intervention. Medical therapy typically emphasizes aqueous suppressants rather than outflow enhancers, given the mechanical nature of the outflow obstruction. Surgical intervention often employs tube shunt procedures rather than trabeculectomy due to the inflammatory nature of the underlying disease and increased risk of restrictive strabismus following limbal surgery. Beyond thyroid eye disease, systemic thyroid dysfunction itself influences glaucoma risk and management. Hypothyroidism has been associated with increased IOP, potentially through reduced aqueous outflow facility and increased hyaluronic acid deposition in the trabecular meshwork. Routine thyroid function screening is warranted in patients with unexplained IOP fluctuations or those requiring escalating therapy without clear cause.

Autoimmune and Rheumatologic Diseases

Autoimmune conditions including rheumatoid arthritis, systemic lupus erythematosus, and seronegative spondyloarthropathies significantly impact glaucoma management through multiple mechanisms. Primary concerns include the increased risk of inflammatory (uveitic) glaucoma, steroid-induced pressure elevation during disease management, and drug-specific ocular side effects. Patients with autoimmune conditions receiving long-term corticosteroid therapy, whether systemic or topical, require regular IOP monitoring and comprehensive glaucoma assessment. Early involvement of glaucoma specialists in cases of steroid-induced pressure elevation allows for coordinated care with rheumatologists, potentially including steroid-sparing immunomodulatory therapy to minimize ocular hypertensive effects while maintaining disease control. Hydroxychloroquine and chloroquine, commonly used in rheumatoid arthritis and lupus, may cause vortex keratopathy that interferes with accurate visual field assessment. These deposits typically do not affect visual function but can complicate monitoring for glaucomatous progression. Medications used in rheumatologic conditions, including non-steroidal anti-inflammatory drugs and certain disease-modifying antirheumatic drugs, can potentially interact with glaucoma medications or influence bleeding risk during glaucoma surgery. Comprehensive medication reconciliation and interdisciplinary communication are essential before surgical intervention in these complex patients.

Neurological Disorders

Neurological conditions may mimic glaucomatous visual field defects, complicating diagnostic assessment. Cerebrovascular disease, compressive lesions affecting the anterior visual pathway, and neurodegenerative disorders can all produce visual field abnormalities that may be confused with or occur concurrently with glaucomatous damage. Patients with unexplained visual field progression despite well-controlled IOP, field defects that respect the vertical rather than horizontal meridian, or disproportionate visual function loss relative to structural findings warrant neuroimaging and neurological evaluation. Conditions such as normal pressure hydrocephalus can cause transient IOP elevations and visual field changes that improve with neurosurgical intervention rather than traditional glaucoma therapy.

From a therapeutic perspective, many medications used in neurological conditions influence glaucoma management. Anticholinergic agents used in Parkinson's disease can precipitate angle closure in susceptible individuals. Topiramate and other sulfa-based anticonvulsants can cause acute angle closure through ciliary body edema and anterior rotation of the lens-iris diaphragm, representing a true ophthalmic emergency requiring prompt recognition and intervention.

To conclude, the management of glaucoma in patients with systemic disease requires comprehensive understanding of potential interactions, coordinated multidisciplinary care, and individualized risk–benefit assessment. Beyond their direct effects on glaucoma pathophysiology, systemic conditions influence treatment options, medication efficacy, surgical outcomes, and overall management priorities. Regular communication between ophthalmologists and other healthcare providers, thorough medication reconciliation, and holistic consideration of the patient's overall health status are essential components of effective glaucoma care in this complex population.

SECTION 4—COST-EFFECTIVE TREATMENTS FOR RESOURCE-LIMITED SETTINGS

Glaucoma represents a significant global health challenge, with approximately 80 million people affected worldwide and more than 90% of glaucoma-related blindness occurring in low- and middle-income countries. Resource-limited settings face substantial barriers to effective glaucoma care, including limited access to specialized equipment, shortage of trained personnel, high medication costs, inadequate follow-up capabilities, and competing healthcare priorities. This section explores pragmatic, evidence-based approaches to glaucoma management in resource-constrained environments, emphasizing cost-effective strategies that maximize visual outcomes within significant economic and infrastructural limitations.

Challenges in Resource-Limited Settings

Several fundamental challenges distinguish glaucoma care in resource-limited settings from that in high-resource environments:

- *Late presentation and advanced disease* characterize the typical glaucoma patient in many low-resource settings, with studies from sub-Saharan Africa and South Asia indicating that 50–70% of patients present with advanced disease affecting at least one eye. This late presentation dramatically reduces treatment options and prognosis, emphasizing the critical need for earlier detection strategies.
- *Limited access to diagnostic equipment* restricts the ability to perform comprehensive glaucoma assessments. Basic technologies like reliable tonometry, visual field testing, and optic nerve imaging remain unavailable in many settings. Clinicians must frequently make management decisions based on limited diagnostic information, prioritizing techniques that provide the most essential clinical data with minimal equipment requirements.
- *Medication cost and availability* present formidable barriers to chronic glaucoma therapy. Brand-name medications remain prohibitively expensive for most patients, while generic alternatives may suffer from quality control issues, limited availability, or restricted selection. Even when medications are subsidized through government programs, supply chain interruptions frequently compromise continuity of care.
- *Surgical resource limitations* include inadequate microsurgical equipment, inconsistent availability of adjunctive agents like antimetabolites, limited operating room access, and insufficient infrastructure for postoperative follow-up. These constraints necessitate surgical approaches that maximize effectiveness while minimizing resource requirements and postoperative complications requiring specialized management.
- *Workforce shortages* represent perhaps the most significant barrier, with extreme scarcity of ophthalmologists, optometrists, and allied eye care professionals

in many regions. Sub-Saharan Africa, for instance, has approximately one ophthalmologist per million population compared to 60–80 per million in high-income countries. This shortage necessitates task-shifting approaches and strategic deployment of the limited specialist workforce.

Practical Approaches to Diagnosis

Diagnostic strategies in resource-limited settings must balance accuracy with practicality, focusing on essential assessments that guide clinical decision-making while requiring minimal specialized equipment.

- *Tonometry options* range from Goldmann applanation tonometry (the gold standard but requiring a slit lamp and regular calibration) to more portable alternatives. The Tonopen offers reasonable accuracy with minimal maintenance requirements, while rebound tonometers like the iCare provide rapid measurements without requiring topical anesthesia, potentially enabling use by non-specialist personnel. In extremely limited settings, Schiotz tonometry, despite its limitations, provides basic pressure assessment with minimal cost. The least resource-intensive option, digital palpation, demonstrates significant variability but can identify grossly elevated pressures when performed by experienced clinicians.
- *Optic nerve examination* remains essential even in the most resource-constrained settings. Direct ophthalmoscopy, while limited by its narrow field of view, provides basic assessment of the cup-to-disc ratio and neuroretinal rim when performed through a dilated pupil. Portable fundus cameras, including smartphone-based systems, increasingly offer affordable options for documenting optic nerve appearance without requiring expensive slit lamps or indirect ophthalmoscopy skills.
- *Visual field assessment*, when automated perimetry is unavailable, may utilize confrontation techniques or manual kinetic perimetry using objects of various sizes against contrasting backgrounds. While significantly less sensitive than automated methods, these approaches can identify moderate to severe field defects that influence management decisions. Tablet-based suprathreshold testing applications offer promising alternatives that balance affordability with improved standardization.

Medication Selection and Access

Pharmacologic management in resource-limited settings emphasizes maximizing effectiveness and adherence while minimizing cost and supply chain vulnerabilities.

- *Prostaglandin analogs*, particularly generic latanoprost, increasingly represent first-line therapy due to once-daily dosing, relatively favorable side effect profile, and falling costs as more generics enter markets worldwide. However, availability and affordability remain inconsistent across regions. Temperature stability concerns in areas without reliable refrigeration may compromise effectiveness, though room temperature stability has been demonstrated for up to 45 days for some formulations.

- *Beta-blockers*, especially generic timolol, remain the most widely available and affordable glaucoma medications globally. Twice-daily dosing represents a disadvantage compared to prostaglandin analogs, but cost differentials often outweigh this consideration in severely resource-constrained settings. The significant contraindications in patients with respiratory and cardiac conditions require careful consideration, particularly when detailed medical history and diagnostic testing are limited.
- *Fixed-combination preparations*, while initially more expensive, may prove cost-effective by improving adherence, reducing preservative exposure, and minimizing the total number of bottles required. Combinations containing low-cost components like timolol with either a carbonic anhydrase inhibitor or alpha-agonist provide reasonable alternatives when prostaglandin analogs are unavailable or unaffordable.
- *Medication access programs* through partnerships between pharmaceutical companies, nongovernmental organizations, and local health systems have successfully increased access to glaucoma medications in some regions. The World Health Organization's inclusion of timolol and, more recently, latanoprost in its Essential Medicines List has facilitated greater availability through government procurement systems. Community-based medication banks and revolving drug funds provide additional models for sustaining access in areas with limited healthcare infrastructure.

Surgical Approaches

In many resource-limited settings, surgical intervention represents not the last resort but rather the most practical approach to preventing blindness from glaucoma, particularly given the challenges of lifelong medical therapy. Ideal surgical procedures in these contexts maximize effectiveness while minimizing equipment requirements, postoperative complications, and follow-up burden. Trabeculectomy remains the most widely performed glaucoma procedure globally and can be completed with basic microsurgical equipment. Modifications for resource-limited settings include using 10–0 nylon sutures (more widely available than releasable or adjustable options), fornix-based conjunctival flaps (technically easier with fewer sutures required), and judicious use of available antimetabolites. When commercial mitomycin C is unavailable, some centers utilize alternatives such as 5-fluorouracil, though requiring multiple injections with their associated complications. A study in Ghana demonstrated good efficacy of trabeculectomy without antimetabolites in African eyes with advanced glaucoma, with 80% maintaining IOP below 21 mmHg at five years (62).

Minimally invasive glaucoma surgery (MIGS) devices, while increasingly popular in high-resource settings, generally remain impractical in resource-limited environments due to high device costs, specialized equipment requirements, and limited efficacy in advanced disease. However, non-device-dependent MIGS procedures such as ab interno trabeculotomy techniques may eventually provide viable options as instrumentation becomes more widely available.

Combined cataract and glaucoma surgery offers particular advantages in resource-limited settings where patients may have a single opportunity for surgical intervention.

While combined procedures demonstrate somewhat higher complication rates than sequential approaches, the balance of risks versus benefits favors a single intervention when follow-up cannot be guaranteed. Manual small-incision cataract surgery combined with trabeculectomy has been successfully implemented in many regions with limited phacoemulsification access.

Transscleral cyclophotocoagulation, particularly using diode laser, offers a non-incisional option with minimal equipment requirements beyond the laser unit itself. In settings where microsurgical facilities are unavailable, appropriately selected cyclophotocoagulation provides effective pressure reduction, though with risks of inflammation, hypotony, and vision loss. Modifications including reduced energy settings and treating fewer clock hours per session can mitigate complications while maintaining efficacy.

Delivery Models and Systems Approaches

Beyond specific clinical interventions, innovative care delivery models offer solutions for extending limited resources to serve larger populations.

For example, task-shifting involves training mid-level eye care personnel in specific aspects of glaucoma care, including screening, basic diagnostic techniques, medication administration education, and routine follow-up. Evidence from several regions demonstrates that appropriately trained ophthalmic nurses, optometrists, and community health workers can effectively perform many aspects of glaucoma management, reserving ophthalmologist involvement for surgical decision-making and intervention.

Teleophthalmology approaches, including remote interpretation of optic nerve photographs and structured patient data, allow extension of specialist expertise to underserved areas. Simple protocols using smartphone photography with security-compliant messaging applications have been successfully implemented in several regions, providing timely specialist input despite geographic barriers. Integrated Eye Care models embedding glaucoma services within comprehensive eye care systems optimize resource utilization. Programs initially developed for cataract or refractive error can incorporate basic glaucoma assessment, creating efficient referral pathways for patients requiring specialized intervention while managing stable patients at community levels.

While resource limitations create significant challenges for glaucoma care, pragmatic approaches emphasizing early detection, strategic resource allocation, and context-appropriate interventions can substantially reduce preventable blindness. Rather than attempting to replicate high-resource models with financial and infrastructural requirements beyond reach, successful programs adapt evidence-based principles to local realities, prioritizing interventions with the greatest population impact given available resources. Through continued innovation in diagnostic techniques, medication delivery, surgical approaches, and care systems, the global burden of glaucoma-related blindness can be progressively reduced even in the most resource-constrained environments.

CHAPTER 9
PUBLIC HEALTH
AND GLAUCOMA

Glaucoma represents a significant global public health challenge, affecting approximately 80 million people worldwide and ranking as the second leading cause of blindness globally. Unlike many other causes of vision loss, glaucoma-related blindness is largely preventable through early detection and appropriate intervention, yet an estimated 50–90% of cases remain undiagnosed in various populations. This disconnect between the availability of effective interventions and the persistent burden of glaucoma-related visual impairment underscores the critical importance of approaching glaucoma not only as a clinical condition but as a public health priority requiring population-level strategies.

The public health dimensions of glaucoma extend far beyond the clinical management of individual patients. They encompass the systematic efforts needed to raise awareness, improve access to care, leverage technological innovations, and address the complex sociocultural factors that influence eye health behaviors across diverse populations. A comprehensive public health approach to glaucoma necessitates coordinated action across multiple sectors, including healthcare systems, community organizations, policymakers, and educational institutions.

This chapter explores four essential aspects of the public health approach to glaucoma. First, we examine awareness campaigns and early detection strategies, recognizing that public knowledge about glaucoma remains inadequate in many communities, limiting opportunities for timely intervention. Second, we address the pervasive disparities in access to glaucoma care, particularly among underserved populations, and explore innovative approaches to bridging these gaps. Third, we investigate the transformative potential of telemedicine and emerging technologies to extend specialized care beyond traditional clinical settings. Finally, we consider how cultural perspectives and socioeconomic factors influence glaucoma diagnosis, treatment adherence, and outcomes across diverse global contexts. By examining these public health dimensions, this chapter aims to complement the clinical focus of previous chapters, highlighting the broader societal and systemic approaches needed to effectively address the global challenge of glaucoma-related vision loss.

SECTION I—AWARENESS CAMPAIGNS AND EARLY DETECTION

The silent, progressive nature of glaucoma presents a fundamental public health challenge: most affected individuals remain asymptomatic until substantial,

DOI: 10.1201/9781003646693-9

irreversible damage has occurred. This characteristic, combined with limited public understanding of the disease, results in late presentation and missed opportunities for vision preservation. Effective awareness campaigns and strategic early detection programs represent essential components of a comprehensive public health approach to reducing glaucoma-related visual impairment. This section examines evidence-based strategies for increasing public knowledge about glaucoma and implementing successful early detection initiatives across diverse populations and settings.

Despite glaucoma's prevalence and significant impact on quality of life, public awareness remains inadequately low worldwide. Multiple studies across various regions and demographic groups consistently demonstrate limited knowledge regarding glaucoma risk factors, symptoms, and the importance of regular screening. A comprehensive systematic review (9) examining global awareness of glaucoma found that only 13–51% of study participants across various countries were aware of glaucoma as a disease that could cause blindness. More concerning, detailed knowledge about risk factors, symptoms, and screening recommendations was substantially lower, ranging from 5–22% across studies.

The consequences of this awareness gap are profound. Limited knowledge contributes to delayed care-seeking, reduced participation in screening programs, and poor adherence to treatment regimens. These factors collectively result in higher rates of advanced disease at presentation, greater vision loss, and increased economic burden on both individuals and healthcare systems. The elderly, racial and ethnic minorities, those with lower educational attainment, and residents of rural areas consistently demonstrate lower awareness levels, contributing to the disproportionate impact of glaucoma in these populations.

Successful glaucoma awareness campaigns employ multiple complementary approaches tailored to target populations. Several evidence-based strategies have demonstrated effectiveness in various contexts:

- *Mass media campaigns* utilizing television, radio, print media, and increasingly, social media platforms, can reach large audiences with key prevention messages. The most effective campaigns employ clear, consistent messaging focused on a limited number of actionable points rather than comprehensive disease education. Messages emphasizing glaucoma's asymptomatic nature, the irreversibility of vision loss, and the effectiveness of early detection resonate particularly well across diverse audiences. Complementing factual information with personal testimonials from affected individuals increases emotional engagement and message retention. The timing and placement of messages warrant careful consideration, with health communication research suggesting that integration into existing programming (rather than standalone public service announcements) and sustained messaging over time yield superior outcomes compared to short-term, high-intensity campaigns.
- *Community-based outreach programs* leverage existing social networks and trusted community institutions to disseminate information and promote screening participation. Successful models include educational sessions in religious institutions, senior centers, and community organizations; health fairs offering information alongside basic screening services; and train-the-trainer approaches that equip community health workers or volunteers with accurate information and communication skills. These interpersonal approaches often prove particularly

effective for reaching underserved populations with limited access to traditional media channels or lower health literacy. Including family members in educational initiatives recognizes their critical role in supporting both screening decisions and treatment adherence, particularly among elderly populations.

- *Educational materials* developed with health literacy principles in mind can effectively supplement other awareness activities. Visual elements including photographs, illustrations, and infographics enhance understanding across literacy levels. Materials should emphasize actionable information, including screening recommendations, risk factors warranting earlier or more frequent assessment, and local resources for eye care. Translation into locally relevant languages and cultural adaptation of content, examples, and imagery improve both comprehension and acceptability. Digital formats, including websites and mobile applications, increasingly complement print materials, particularly for reaching younger populations and those seeking more detailed information following exposure to basic awareness messages.

- *Professional and system-level initiatives* recognize that awareness gaps exist not only among the general public but also among healthcare providers outside ophthalmology. Educational programs targeting primary care physicians, general practitioners, pharmacists, and other frontline healthcare providers can significantly increase appropriate referrals for glaucoma assessment. Incorporating basic glaucoma risk assessment into routine health encounters and electronic health record systems creates additional opportunities for identifying high-risk individuals who would benefit from comprehensive evaluation.

While universal population-based screening for glaucoma has not demonstrated cost-effectiveness in most settings, targeted early detection strategies can significantly reduce the burden of undiagnosed disease. Several approaches warrant consideration:

- *Risk-stratified screening* targets resources toward those at highest risk for glaucoma, including individuals over age 40 with family history of glaucoma, African or Hispanic ancestry, history of ocular trauma or steroid use, and certain systemic conditions like diabetes. This approach improves yield and cost-effectiveness compared to universal age-based screening. Validated risk calculators incorporating multiple factors can further refine risk assessment, though their implementation in routine practice remains limited.

- *Integration with existing health services* leverages established healthcare touchpoints to incorporate glaucoma detection. Examples include adding intraocular pressure screening to diabetic retinopathy assessments, incorporating basic glaucoma evaluation into routine vision care, and implementing opportunistic screening during encounters for other health conditions. The World Glaucoma Association advocates for this integrated approach, particularly in resource-limited settings where standalone glaucoma programs may be impractical.

- *Tiered assessment approaches* balance sensitivity, specificity, and resource utilization through staged evaluation processes. Initial screening using non-specialist personnel and basic equipment (tonometry, optic disc photography, or tablet-based visual field assessment) identifies individuals requiring more comprehensive evaluation by specialists with advanced diagnostic capabilities.

This approach extends limited specialist resources while maximizing population coverage. A large-scale implementation (63) indicated the feasibility and effectiveness of this approach using smartphone-based tools for initial assessment followed by specialist referral, identifying previously undetected glaucoma cases in remote communities with minimal ophthalmic infrastructure.

- *Telehealth integration* enables remote interpretation of diagnostic information collected in community settings by trained technicians. Digital imaging of the optic nerve, along with structured data collection regarding risk factors and basic examination findings, allows specialist review without requiring patient travel to tertiary centers. This approach proves particularly valuable in rural and underserved urban areas with limited specialist access.

Evaluating awareness and early detection initiatives requires thoughtfully selected metrics that capture both process and outcome measures. Comprehensive assessment includes the following:

- *Knowledge and awareness metrics* measure changes in public understanding using standardized instruments administered before and after campaigns. Beyond simple disease recognition, these assessments should evaluate understanding of risk factors, screening recommendations, and the importance of early detection.
- *Behavioral metrics* track changes in screening participation, care-seeking patterns, and adherence to follow-up recommendations. These intermediate outcomes provide early indication of campaign effectiveness before long-term clinical outcomes become apparent.
- *Clinical outcome metrics* such as stage of disease at diagnosis, proportion of cases detected before significant visual field loss, and rates of glaucoma-related vision impairment represent the ultimate measures of program success. However, these outcomes typically require longer timeframes and more complex data systems to evaluate effectively.
- *Economic metrics* including cost per case detected, cost per quality-adjusted life year gained, and broader economic impacts provide essential information for policymakers and healthcare systems considering program implementation or expansion.

Continuous quality improvement principles should guide program refinement, with ongoing data collection, regular analysis, and responsive modification of approaches based on performance metrics. Particularly successful are adaptive models that customize messaging and outreach strategies based on community characteristics, gradually focusing resources on approaches demonstrating greatest impact in specific populations.

Effective awareness campaigns and early detection programs represent essential foundations for reducing the public health burden of glaucoma. While significant challenges remain in reaching underserved populations and translating awareness into action, evidence-based approaches combining mass media, community engagement, and integration with existing healthcare services demonstrate promise. As technological innovations expand screening capabilities and communication channels continue to evolve, opportunities for creative, cost-effective interventions will further enhance our ability to identify glaucoma in its earliest, most treatable stages—ultimately reducing preventable vision loss across diverse populations worldwide.

SECTION 2—ACCESS TO CARE IN UNDERSERVED COMMUNITIES

Despite significant advances in glaucoma diagnosis and treatment, substantial disparities persist in access to appropriate care, particularly among underserved populations. These disparities contribute to higher rates of undiagnosed disease, delayed intervention, and ultimately, preventable vision loss in vulnerable communities. Addressing these access barriers requires understanding the different challenges faced by underserved populations and implementing targeted, culturally appropriate solutions that extend beyond traditional care models. This section examines the dimensions of access disparities and explores innovative approaches to expanding glaucoma care for those most at risk.

Access to glaucoma care encompasses multiple interrelated dimensions that extend beyond simple geographic proximity to eye care providers. Comprehensive understanding of these barriers is essential for developing effective interventions:

- *Geographic barriers* represent the most visible access challenge, with significant maldistribution of eye care specialists globally and within countries. Rural populations often face prohibitive travel distances to reach specialists, while underserved urban areas may have numerical proximity to providers but limited actual accessibility due to transportation barriers or provider practices that do not serve certain populations. A comprehensive analysis (64) documented the extreme global disparities in eye care workforce distribution, with high-income countries having up to 83 times more ophthalmologists per population than low-income countries. Even within high-income nations, rural areas and disadvantaged urban communities frequently demonstrate significant provider shortages.

- *Financial barriers* include direct costs of care (consultation fees, diagnostic testing, and medication expenses) and indirect costs (transportation, lost wages, and childcare expenses associated with seeking care). In countries without universal health coverage, insurance status significantly influences access, with uninsured and underinsured individuals less likely to receive regular eye examinations or adhere to recommended glaucoma treatment. Even in settings with national health systems, incomplete coverage of diagnostic tests, medications, or certain surgical procedures creates financial obstacles to comprehensive glaucoma management. For chronic conditions like glaucoma, these costs accumulate over decades, creating substantial financial burden that may lead to discontinued care.

- *Structural barriers* within healthcare systems include fragmented care delivery, complex referral processes, insufficient coordination between primary and specialty care, and inadequate provider time for patient education. Clinical settings with limited language services, inconvenient hours, or lengthy waiting times create additional obstacles, particularly for working individuals or those with family caregiving responsibilities. These systemic challenges disproportionately affect those with limited health literacy, communication barriers, or fewer resources to navigate complex healthcare systems.

- *Cultural and knowledge barriers* influence both care-seeking behavior and engagement with recommended treatment. Limited awareness of glaucoma's asymptomatic nature, misconceptions about treatment necessity, and cultural beliefs regarding vision loss as an inevitable consequence of aging may all reduce proactive eye care utilization. Additionally, mistrust of healthcare systems based on historical injustices or negative experiences affects willingness to engage with care, particularly among certain racial and ethnic minorities.
- *Provider-level factors* include unconscious bias, communication challenges with patients from different cultural backgrounds, and limited cultural competence in clinical interactions. These factors can result in lower quality care, reduced patient satisfaction, and ultimately, decreased adherence to treatment recommendations. Clinical settings that fail to represent the diversity of the communities they serve may further exacerbate these challenges through limited cultural understanding and perspective.

Addressing these multidimensional access barriers requires innovative approaches that extend beyond traditional care models. Several promising strategies demonstrate potential for expanding glaucoma care in underserved communities:

- *Task-shifting and workforce expansion* leverage non-specialist personnel to extend the reach of limited specialist resources. Various models have been successfully implemented, including training primary care physicians, optometrists, or community health workers to perform basic glaucoma screening and monitoring. Well-designed protocols, appropriate training, and clear referral pathways allow these personnel to identify high-risk individuals and those requiring specialist evaluation while managing stable patients under specialist supervision. This approach has demonstrated particular success in settings with severe specialist shortages, though implementation requires addressing scope-of-practice regulations, establishing appropriate quality assurance mechanisms, and ensuring adequate training and supervision.
- *Mobile outreach programs* may bring diagnostic capabilities directly to underserved communities through specially equipped vehicles or temporary clinics in community settings. These programs reduce geographic and transportation barriers while leveraging community trust in familiar settings. While traditionally focused on screening, increasingly sophisticated portable equipment enables more comprehensive assessment, including tonometry, visual field testing, and digital imaging for remote interpretation. The integration of electronic health records and telehealth capabilities allows continuity between outreach activities and follow-up care. Successful implementations balance the breadth of population coverage with the depth of services provided, often employing risk stratification to determine appropriate evaluation intensity for each individual.
- *Telehealth applications* can enable remote evaluation of glaucoma-related data collected by trained technicians in community settings. Asynchronous models, where specialist review occurs separately from data collection, maximize efficiency and extend specialist capacity. Clinical validation studies demonstrate good agreement between in-person and telehealth-based assessments for many aspects of glaucoma evaluation, including optic nerve assessment via digital imaging, interpretation

of visual field results, and management decision-making based on structured data collection. Implementation challenges include ensuring adequate image quality, establishing appropriate reimbursement mechanisms, addressing licensure restrictions, and developing protocols for timely management of urgent findings.

- *Integrated care models* embed glaucoma services within other healthcare activities to leverage existing touchpoints with the healthcare system. Examples include incorporating glaucoma assessment into diabetic retinopathy screening programs, integrating basic evaluation into primary care settings serving high-risk populations, and co-locating services with other community-based health programs. These approaches reduce the burden of multiple appointments, minimize transportation barriers, and potentially increase participation by connecting glaucoma care with services patients may perceive as more immediately necessary.

- *Community health worker programs* employ trusted individuals from the community to serve as bridges between formal healthcare systems and underserved populations. These workers provide education, assist with navigating complex healthcare systems, support adherence to treatment regimens, and help overcome logistical barriers to care. Their effectiveness stems from cultural concordance, established community relationships, and understanding of local barriers and facilitators to care. For glaucoma specifically, community health workers can reinforce the importance of ongoing treatment despite absence of symptoms, assist with proper medication administration, and facilitate regular follow-up appointments.

- *Medication access programs* address the financial barriers to ongoing treatment through various mechanisms, including pharmaceutical company patient assistance programs, nonprofit medication banks, and government subsidy initiatives. Given the chronic nature of glaucoma therapy, sustainable approaches must extend beyond short-term solutions to ensure continuous medication access throughout the disease course. Formulary decisions at health system and governmental levels significantly impact treatment affordability, with inclusion of effective, low-cost medications like generic prostaglandin analogs and beta-blockers being particularly important for expanding access.

Successful implementation of access expansion initiatives requires attention to several key factors as listed here:

- *Community engagement* throughout program development and implementation ensures relevance, acceptability, and sustainability. Community advisory boards, focus groups, and partnerships with trusted community organizations provide essential insights into local barriers and potential solutions. Programs developed in collaboration with the communities they serve demonstrate higher participation rates and greater sustainability than those imposed without meaningful community input.

- *Cultural competence* in all aspects of program design and delivery enhances effectiveness across diverse populations. This includes linguistic appropriateness, respect for cultural beliefs and practices, and recognition of historical contexts that may influence trust in healthcare systems. Materials, messaging, and service delivery approaches should reflect the specific needs and preferences of target communities rather than simply translating or transferring approaches developed for majority populations.

Table 9.1 Barriers to Glaucoma Care in Low-Resource Settings

Barrier	Explanation	Proposed Solution
Lack of Awareness	Patients unaware of disease	Community education programs
Cost of Medications	Limited affordability	Generic drugs, subsidies
Scarcity of Specialists	Rural and remote areas	Teleophthalmology, task-shifting
Poor Follow-Up Rates	Non-adherence due to travel or cost	Mobile clinics, simplified regimens

- *Sustainability planning* from initial program development ensures long-term impact beyond grant cycles or initial implementation periods. This includes developing diverse funding streams, building local capacity through training and mentorship, integrating with existing healthcare infrastructure, and demonstrating value to healthcare systems through rigorous evaluation of both clinical and economic outcomes.
- *Health policy advocacy* addresses systemic barriers that impede access to glaucoma care. Priorities include expanding insurance coverage for glaucoma services, ensuring adequate reimbursement for preventive care, reducing regulatory barriers to telehealth implementation, and supporting scope-of-practice expansions that enable greater involvement of non-ophthalmologist providers in appropriate aspects of glaucoma care. Table 9.1 outlines the main barriers to effective glaucoma care in low-resource and underserved settings. It further suggests targeted strategies to address these challenges, reflecting the growing need for context-sensitive solutions in global glaucoma management.

Improving access to glaucoma care for underserved populations requires comprehensive understanding of the multidimensional barriers these communities face and implementation of targeted, culturally appropriate solutions. While significant challenges remain, innovative approaches including task-shifting, mobile outreach, telehealth applications, and community-based programs demonstrate promising results in expanding access to this sight-saving care. As these models continue to evolve and scale, their potential to reduce disparities in glaucoma outcomes offers hope for more equitable eye health across diverse populations and settings.

SECTION 3—THE ROLE OF TELEMEDICINE AND TECHNOLOGY

The convergence of technological innovation, digital connectivity, and healthcare delivery models has created unprecedented opportunities to transform glaucoma care. Telemedicine and emerging technologies offer promising solutions to longstanding challenges in glaucoma management, including access limitations, monitoring difficulties, adherence barriers, and workforce shortages. These approaches are increasingly moving from experimental innovations to practical tools with demonstrated clinical utility. This section examines the current state and future potential of telemedicine and technology in addressing the public health burden of glaucoma, with emphasis on validated applications, implementation considerations, and emerging directions.

Teleglaucoma: Models and Evidence

Teleglaucoma encompasses various models for remote glaucoma assessment, ranging from basic screening applications to comprehensive management programs. Several models have demonstrated clinical validity and utility:

- *Store-and-forward teleglaucoma* involves capturing clinical data (digital images, visual field results, tonometry readings) at remote locations by trained technicians, with subsequent asynchronous interpretation by specialists. This approach allows extension of specialist expertise without requiring simultaneous presence of patient and provider. The data collection sites may include primary care clinics, optometry practices, mobile screening units, or community health centers. A systematic review and meta-analysis (65) found that store-and-forward teleglaucoma demonstrated 83% sensitivity and 79% specificity for glaucoma detection when compared to in-person comprehensive examination, with greater cost-effectiveness in high-risk populations and remote settings. This approach has proven particularly valuable for screening and triage, identifying patients requiring in-person specialist evaluation while avoiding unnecessary referrals for those with normal findings.

- *Remote monitoring applications* enable ongoing assessment of disease stability between office visits through home-based testing, data collection, and transmission to providers. These applications range from smartphone-based visual field tests and virtual reality perimetry systems to home tonometry devices and medication adherence monitoring tools. Integration of these various data streams creates comprehensive remote monitoring systems that may detect disease progression or treatment failure earlier than traditional episodic in-office evaluations. A study (66) showed that home IOP monitoring combined with virtual provider review identified significant pressure fluctuations and treatment inefficacy not captured during standard office visits, leading to earlier treatment modifications and improved pressure control.

- *Virtual glaucoma clinics* combine remote data acquisition with structured assessment protocols, enabling efficient evaluation of stable glaucoma patients without direct specialist involvement in every encounter. In these models, technicians collect comprehensive data including imaging, visual fields, and tonometry. Specialists review results through electronic systems, identifying patients requiring in-person evaluation while providing management recommendations for those with stable disease. Well-designed protocols establish clear criteria for distinguishing routine from concerning findings. This approach significantly expands specialist capacity while maintaining quality care, with studies demonstrating non-inferiority to traditional models for stable patients. Implementation considerations include appropriate patient selection, quality assurance mechanisms, and clear protocols for managing unexpected findings or acute concerns.

- *Direct-to-patient telemedicine* connects patients and providers through synchronous video consultations. While limited in ability to perform comprehensive glaucoma evaluation, this approach facilitates medication management, addresses patient questions, and provides continuity between in-person assessments. The COVID-19 pandemic accelerated adoption of these models, with many practices developing hybrid approaches combining remote consultation with in-person testing. Guidelines from professional organizations now provide frameworks for appropriate utilization of direct video consultation in glaucoma care, including patient selection criteria and recommended frequency of in-person evaluation.

Several technological innovations serve as foundational elements enabling effective teleglaucoma implementation:

- *Remote-capable imaging devices* provide high-quality visualization of ocular structures without requiring specialist operation. Non-mydriatic fundus cameras with increasing resolution and field-of-view capabilities enable detailed optic nerve assessment through undilated pupils, enhancing patient comfort and deployment feasibility. Smartphone-based fundus photography adaptors significantly reduce equipment costs while maintaining adequate image quality for screening purposes. Anterior segment imaging devices document angle configuration and other structures relevant to glaucoma diagnosis and classification. Cloud-based storage and transmission systems facilitate image sharing between acquisition sites and interpretation centers, with appropriate security protocols to ensure patient confidentiality.

- *Portable and automated tonometry* addresses the challenge of measuring intraocular pressure outside traditional clinical settings. Rebound tonometers like the iCare HOME enable patient self-monitoring with reasonable accuracy compared to Goldmann applanation tonometry, though individual correlation should be established before relying on home readings for management decisions. Continuous monitoring devices, though still evolving, show promise for capturing diurnal fluctuations and treatment effects with greater precision than isolated measurements. These devices increasingly incorporate automated data transmission capabilities, eliminating manual recording errors and facilitating integration with electronic health records.

- *Alternative perimetry platforms* adapt traditional visual field testing for telehealth applications. Tablet-based suprathreshold strategies demonstrate reasonable correlation with standard automated perimetry while requiring minimal equipment and technical expertise. Virtual reality perimetric testing using head-mounted displays provides standardized testing environments regardless of ambient conditions, potentially enabling home-based assessment. While these alternative platforms may not yet replace standard clinical perimetry for definitive diagnosis, they offer valuable screening and monitoring capabilities in telehealth contexts. Continued refinement of testing algorithms and validation studies are gradually narrowing the performance gap between traditional and alternative platforms.

- *Artificial intelligence applications* enhance multiple aspects of teleglaucoma implementation. Automated image analysis systems can identify key glaucomatous features in fundus photographs and OCT scans with sensitivity and specificity approaching expert human assessment. These systems enable preliminary interpretation at the point of image acquisition, supporting appropriate triage decisions. Additionally, AI algorithms integrating multiple data sources (imaging, visual fields, risk factors) can generate risk assessments and progression analyses that guide remote management decisions. Pattern recognition capabilities identify subtle progression not readily apparent through conventional analysis, potentially enabling earlier intervention. While these technologies do not replace specialist judgment, they extend capabilities of non-specialist personnel and enhance efficiency of specialist review processes.

Successful teleglaucoma implementation requires attention to several key factors beyond the technological components:

- *Validation and quality assurance* mechanisms ensure clinical effectiveness comparable to traditional care models. This includes validation of equipment performance against gold standards, establishment of image quality standards with processes for managing inadequate studies, ongoing monitoring of diagnostic accuracy, and regular calibration of devices. Systematic comparison of telehealth assessments with periodic in-person evaluations provides essential quality verification, particularly for chronic management applications where subtle progression may influence treatment decisions.
- *Workflow integration* determines practical feasibility in routine clinical environments. Successful implementation minimizes disruption to existing processes while addressing inefficiencies in traditional models. Electronic health record integration enables seamless documentation and communication between remote sites and interpretation centers. Clear protocols for managing abnormal findings, technical failures, and urgent situations ensure appropriate escalation when needed. Staff roles require explicit definition, with adequate training for those acquiring data and interpreting results.
- *Economic considerations* significantly influence sustainability and scalability. Initial implementation costs include equipment acquisition, staff training, connectivity infrastructure, and workflow redesign. Ongoing expenses encompass maintenance, technical support, and personnel time. These investments must be balanced against benefits including increased patient capacity, reduced travel requirements, more efficient specialist utilization, and potential earlier detection of disease progression. Reimbursement mechanisms vary substantially across healthcare systems, with some regions developing specific teleglaucoma payment models while others require adapting existing reimbursement structures. Full economic evaluation should consider both direct healthcare costs and broader societal benefits including reduced vision loss, decreased caregiver burden, and maintained workforce participation.
- *Regulatory and legal frameworks* continue to evolve alongside telehealth technologies. Issues requiring consideration include licensure requirements for providers delivering care across geographic boundaries, liability coverage for telehealth activities, data privacy and security regulations, and informed consent processes specifically addressing telehealth components. Many regions implemented temporary regulatory accommodations during the COVID-19 pandemic, creating natural experiments that inform development of permanent frameworks balancing access expansion with appropriate quality standards.

Evident from the developments described previously, the teleglaucoma landscape continues to evolve with several promising technologies on the horizon:

- *Home-based OCT devices* currently under development would enable remote assessment of retinal nerve fiber layer and ganglion cell complex thickness, providing objective structural measurements currently requiring office visits. While these systems likely will not immediately match the resolution and precision of clinical devices, their potential for frequent longitudinal assessment could enable earlier detection of progressive changes despite somewhat lower absolute accuracy.

- *Continuous IOP monitoring systems* incorporated into contact lenses, intraocular implants, or external devices promise more comprehensive pressure assessment than isolated measurements. These technologies could fundamentally transform our understanding of pressure fluctuations and their relationship to disease progression while enabling precise titration of therapeutic interventions. Early validation studies demonstrate encouraging correlation with reference standard measurements, though long-term safety, stability, and clinical utility require further investigation.

- *Integrated remote monitoring ecosystems* combining multiple data streams (structural imaging, functional testing, IOP, medication adherence) with patient-reported outcomes create comprehensive digital phenotyping platforms. These systems potentially enable highly personalized risk assessment and treatment adjustment based on individual patterns rather than population averages. The wealth of longitudinal data generated through these approaches, when aggregated and analyzed appropriately, may yield insights into disease mechanisms and treatment response patterns not apparent through traditional research methodologies.

- *Automated intervention systems* represent the logical extension of remote monitoring capabilities. These systems would implement algorithm-driven interventions (e.g., medication adjustments, appointment scheduling) based on predefined parameters and provider-approved protocols, enabling more responsive management without requiring direct provider action for every decision. Patient-facing components would provide context-appropriate education and support based on monitored parameters and identified challenges. While raising important questions regarding autonomy, liability, and the fundamental nature of the provider–patient relationship, these systems hold promise for more dynamic management approaches than current episodic models permit.

Figure 9.1 presents a schematic illustration of benefits of different applications in glaucoma as discussed in this section.

To conclude, telemedicine and technology applications in glaucoma care have rapidly evolved from theoretical possibilities to practical tools with demonstrated clinical utility. When thoughtfully implemented with appropriate validation, quality assurance, and integration into care delivery systems, these approaches can significantly expand access, enhance monitoring precision, improve efficiency, and potentially transform management paradigms. While traditional in-person comprehensive examination remains essential for certain aspects of glaucoma care, the judicious incorporation of telehealth components creates hybrid models that leverage the strengths of both approaches. As technologies continue to advance and

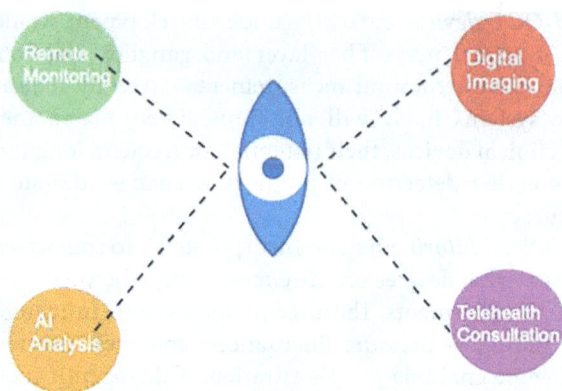

Benefits: Improved Access • Early Detection • Continuous Monitoring • Reduced Travel

Figure 9.1 Benefits of different application in glaucoma.

implementation experience grows, teleglaucoma will likely become an increasingly integral component of public health strategies to reduce the burden of glaucoma-related visual impairment

SECTION 4—CULTURAL PERSPECTIVES ON EYE CARE

The experience of glaucoma—from risk perception and symptom interpretation to treatment decisions and management adherence—is profoundly influenced by cultural context and socioeconomic realities. Understanding these influences is essential for developing effective public health approaches that resonate with diverse populations and address the complex barriers to optimal eye care. This section examines how cultural beliefs, socioeconomic factors, and health system contexts shape glaucoma outcomes globally, with emphasis on their implications for culturally responsive interventions and policy approaches.

Cultural frameworks fundamentally shape how individuals conceptualize health, illness, and appropriate care-seeking behaviors. Several aspects of cultural understanding particularly influence glaucoma care:

- *Explanatory models of eye disease* vary substantially across cultural contexts, influencing how symptoms are interpreted and when care is sought. In many communities, vision changes are attributed to natural aging processes rather than pathological conditions requiring intervention. Research in diverse settings has documented attribution of visual symptoms to factors including spiritual causes, environmental exposures, dietary imbalances, or violation of cultural taboos. These interpretations may delay medical consultation until symptoms become severe, particularly when traditional or cultural healing practices represent the first line of response to vision changes. In some contexts, the concept of asymptomatic disease requiring treatment conflicts with cultural frameworks that define illness primarily through experienced symptoms, creating challenges for preventive care and early intervention.

- *Cultural attitudes toward prevention* significantly influence engagement with screening and early detection programs. Societies with strong future orientation and emphasis on prevention generally demonstrate greater participation in screening activities, while those with present-focused temporal orientation may prioritize more immediate health concerns. Fatalistic perspectives regarding health outcomes—the belief that disease and disability represent inevitable fate rather than preventable conditions—correlate with reduced preventive behaviors across multiple health domains including eye care. These attitudes are often reinforced through community narratives about vision loss as an expected consequence of aging or particular lifestyles.

- *Family and community roles* in health decision-making vary across cultural contexts, with significant implications for glaucoma care. In collectivist societies, health decisions frequently involve extended family networks rather than representing individual choices. Recognition of these decision-making structures is essential when designing educational interventions and obtaining meaningful consent for treatment. The role of family members in supporting treatment adherence takes different forms across cultures, ranging from direct supervision of medication administration to provision of transportation and financial support. Engaging these support networks appropriately requires understanding their structure and function within specific cultural contexts.

Moreover, socioeconomic factors profoundly influence glaucoma outcomes through multiple pathways that extend beyond simple financial barriers.

- *Educational disparities* affect health literacy, symptom recognition, and ability to navigate complex healthcare systems. Lower educational attainment correlates with reduced knowledge about glaucoma and its risk factors, decreased recognition of the importance of regular screening, and greater difficulty understanding treatment instructions. These associations persist across diverse geographic and cultural settings, though their magnitude varies based on healthcare system structure and communication approaches. Educational interventions must account for these disparities through appropriate literacy levels, visual communication methods, and reinforcement of key concepts rather than assuming baseline knowledge.

- *Economic constraints* extend beyond direct costs of care to encompass complex opportunity costs and resource allocation decisions. For individuals with limited economic resources, particularly in settings without robust social safety nets, seeking preventive eye care may represent sacrificing immediate necessities. The chronic nature of glaucoma creates particular challenges, as treatment costs accumulate over decades while benefits remain largely preventive rather than restorative. These economic realities necessitate structural solutions beyond individual education or behavior change approaches. A review study (67) examining barriers to cataract surgery in low- and middle-income countries identified direct and indirect costs as the most frequently reported barriers across diverse settings, with findings applicable to other chronic eye conditions including glaucoma.

- *Gender disparities* in glaucoma care access and outcomes manifest differently across cultural contexts but consistently disadvantage women in most settings. These disparities result from multiple factors including lower financial autonomy, greater caregiving responsibilities limiting healthcare access, reduced educational opportunities affecting health literacy, and gender-based differences in healthcare-seeking authorization within family structures. Additionally, in some contexts, women's health concerns receive lower priority in family resource allocation decisions. Addressing these disparities requires gender-sensitive approaches that consider both practical barriers to care and underlying structural inequities.

Developing culturally responsive approaches to glaucoma care requires moving beyond simple translation of materials or superficial cultural adaptations to engage meaningfully with diverse worldviews and contexts:

- *Culturally adapted communication* involves tailoring messages about glaucoma risk, prevention, and treatment to align with cultural frameworks and values. Effective adaptation goes beyond language translation to incorporate culturally resonant metaphors, examples, and visual representations. Messages emphasizing family responsibility rather than individual health may prove more compelling in collectivist cultures, while those highlighting autonomy and self-determination may better motivate behavior in individualistic contexts. Communication channels require similar cultural alignment, with recognition that trusted information sources vary substantially across communities.
- *Integration with traditional healing systems* offers potential for more comprehensive and culturally acceptable care models in many settings. Rather than positioning biomedical and traditional approaches as oppositional, collaborative models acknowledge the important role of traditional healers as community health authorities while ensuring patients receive effective medical interventions. Various integration approaches have demonstrated success, from formal referral relationships between traditional healers and eye care professionals to incorporation of cultural healing practices into mainstream clinical settings when compatible with medical treatment. These approaches recognize that patients frequently navigate multiple healing systems simultaneously rather than choosing exclusively between traditional and biomedical care.
- *Trust building and historical context* require acknowledgment of past injustices and negative experiences that may influence engagement with healthcare systems. In many communities, particularly those with histories of marginalization or exploitation, mistrust of medical institutions represents a rational response to historical experience rather than simple misunderstanding requiring correction. Addressing this mistrust necessitates both systemic changes in healthcare delivery and interpersonal approaches emphasizing respect, transparency, and

cultural humility. Community partnerships, involvement of trusted cultural brokers, and visible diversity within eye care professions all contribute to building trust in historically marginalized communities.

The broader health system environment fundamentally shapes how cultural and socioeconomic factors influence glaucoma outcomes:

- *Health system organization* determines how cultural factors interact with care delivery models. Vertically organized programs focusing exclusively on eye care may achieve technical efficiency but often fail to integrate with cultural contexts and community priorities. Horizontally integrated approaches embedding eye care within primary healthcare systems typically demonstrate greater cultural accessibility but may sacrifice specialized expertise. Diagonal approaches combining elements of both models show promise for balancing specialized care with cultural responsiveness. The relative effectiveness of these models varies substantially based on specific cultural contexts, existing healthcare infrastructure, and workforce availability.
- *Policy approaches* to addressing cultural and socioeconomic barriers range from targeted interventions to structural reforms. Targeted approaches include cultural competence training for providers, development of culturally adapted educational materials, and community health worker programs employing individuals from the cultures being served. Structural approaches address underlying determinants through health insurance reforms reducing financial barriers, educational initiatives enhancing health literacy, transportation infrastructure improvements, and workforce diversity policies. Comprehensive strategies typically require components addressing both immediate barriers and fundamental determinants.

In summary, cultural perspectives and socioeconomic realities profoundly influence every aspect of glaucoma care, from risk perception and diagnosis to treatment decisions and long-term management. Effective public health approaches must engage meaningfully with these factors, moving beyond simplistic views of "compliance" toward nuanced understanding of how diverse cultural frameworks shape the experience of eye health and illness. By developing interventions and policies that respond to both cultural contexts and socioeconomic realities, we can work toward more equitable glaucoma outcomes across diverse global populations.

CHAPTER 10
CASE STUDIES IN GLAUCOMA

The management of glaucoma, while guided by evidence-based principles and standardized protocols, frequently requires nuanced clinical judgment that extends beyond textbook descriptions. The complexity and heterogeneity of this disease demand an approach that balances scientific rigor with adaptive problem-solving and individualized care. Case studies provide a valuable bridge between theoretical knowledge and practical application, offering insights into the critical thinking processes that distinguish expert clinical practice. This chapter presents a collection of challenging and instructive cases that illuminate the art of glaucoma management across various clinical scenarios.

Diagnostic challenges in glaucoma are commonplace, with presentations that often defy straightforward categorization or mimic other conditions. The first section of this chapter examines cases where diagnosis proved particularly challenging, exploring the thought processes, investigative approaches, and differential considerations that ultimately led to correct identification. These retrospective analyses reveal both the pitfalls that can delay proper diagnosis and the creative problem-solving strategies that facilitate accurate assessment in complex presentations.

Surgical management of glaucoma continues to evolve with new technologies and techniques, yet outcomes remain highly variable and sometimes unpredictable. The second section presents unique surgical cases that required customized approaches, innovative modifications of standard techniques, or management of unexpected complications. These cases highlight the decision-making behind surgical planning, the technical considerations during intervention, and the adaptive responses to both successful and suboptimal outcomes.

Even the most experienced clinicians encounter cases that defy conventional management strategies or present with rare combinations of clinical factors. The final section explores complex cases that required integrated approaches spanning medical, surgical, and interdisciplinary care. These cases offer particular value in demonstrating how multiple management strategies can be synthesized to address challenging clinical scenarios and how apparent treatment failures can become valuable learning opportunities. Collectively, these case studies provide a window into the clinical reasoning process that characterizes expert glaucoma management. By examining both successes and challenges, this chapter aims to enhance the reader's ability to approach complex cases systematically, think critically about diagnostic and management dilemmas, and develop the adaptive expertise needed to optimize outcomes across the diverse spectrum of glaucoma presentations

DOI: 10.1201/9781003646693-10

SECTION 1—DIAGNOSTIC CHALLENGES: A RETROSPECTIVE ANALYSIS

Accurate diagnosis forms the foundation of effective glaucoma management, yet this critical first step often presents significant challenges. The heterogeneous nature of glaucoma, overlap with other optic neuropathies, confounding ocular and systemic factors, and limitations of diagnostic technologies all contribute to potential diagnostic uncertainty. This section presents several challenging cases that highlight common diagnostic dilemmas, exploring the clinical reasoning processes, investigative approaches, and lessons learned through retrospective analysis.

Case 10.1.1 The Masquerader—Distinguishing Normal-Tension Glaucoma from Other Optic Neuropathies

---

A 47-year-old female presented with gradually progressive visual field loss in her right eye detected during a routine examination. She had no significant ocular history and reported mild headaches over the past year that were attributed to work-related stress. Initial examination revealed visual acuity of 20/20 in both eyes, intraocular pressures of 17 mmHg OU, and normal anterior segment findings. Optic nerve examination showed right optic disc pallor with superior and temporal rim thinning and a cup-to-disc ratio of 0.7 OD compared to 0.3 OS. Visual field testing demonstrated an inferior arcuate defect respecting the horizontal meridian in the right eye.

The initial diagnosis was normal-tension glaucoma (NTG) based on the characteristic optic nerve appearance and visual field defect despite normal IOP. Treatment was initiated with a prostaglandin analog. At six-month follow-up, the patient reported worsening headaches and slight progression of visual field loss despite a 20% reduction in IOP.

- *Diagnostic Challenge*: The case presented a common clinical dilemma—distinguishing between NTG and other optic neuropathies that can mimic glaucomatous damage. The asymmetry between eyes, relatively young age of onset, and progression despite IOP reduction raised concerns about alternative diagnoses.
- *Investigative Approach*: Additional diagnostic steps included the following:

1. Diurnal IOP measurements, which remained within normal limits
2. OCT imaging showing RNFL thinning in a pattern consistent with the visual field defect
3. Color vision testing, which revealed a subtle red-green defect in the right eye
4. Visual field testing of the left eye, which demonstrated a subtle superior defect not previously noted
5. Careful review of the optic nerve appearance, revealing pallor exceeding cupping

Based on these findings, neuroimaging was ordered. MRI revealed a right-sided compressive lesion of the optic chiasm consistent with a pituitary adenoma. The patient was referred for neurosurgical intervention, which successfully halted further vision loss.

- *Retrospective Analysis*: This case illustrates several important diagnostic principles. First, asymmetric optic nerve damage, particularly with predominant pallor rather than excavation, should prompt consideration of non-glaucomatous optic neuropathy. As emphasized by reviews of differentiating glaucomatous from non-glaucomatous optic neuropathy, pallor exceeding cupping, reduced visual acuity, color vision abnormalities, and visual field defects that respect the vertical rather than horizontal meridian represent important "red flags" warranting further investigation (68).

Second, progression despite adequate IOP reduction should always trigger reassessment of the diagnosis. While NTG can certainly progress despite treatment, rapid progression in a young patient with normal pressures merits particular scrutiny. Finally, the case demonstrates the value of comprehensive diagnostic evaluation before committing to a lifetime of glaucoma therapy, particularly in atypical presentations.

Case 10.1.2   The Confounder—Myopia and Glaucoma Assessment

A 35-year-old male of Romani descent with high myopia (-7.50 diopters OU) was referred for glaucoma evaluation due to suspicious optic nerve appearance noted during a routine examination. He had no family history of glaucoma and no ocular symptoms. Examination revealed visual acuity of 20/20 OU with correction, IOPs of 19 mmHg OU, and normal anterior segment findings including open angles on gonioscopy. Optic nerve examination showed large, tilted discs with temporal peripapillary atrophy, large cups, and apparent thinning of the superotemporal rim OU.

Initial OCT imaging demonstrated "abnormal" retinal nerve fiber layer thinning superiorly in both eyes according to the instrument's normative database. Visual field testing showed scattered defects with poor reliability indices. The referring optometrist had initiated treatment with a prostaglandin analog based on the structural findings and "presumed early glaucomatous damage."

- *Diagnostic Challenge*: This case highlights the substantial difficulty in distinguishing between myopic disc changes and early glaucoma, a common clinical dilemma particularly in Romani populations with high prevalence of myopia. Myopic discs frequently display large cups, tilting, peripapillary atrophy, and RNFL patterns that deviate from normative databases developed primarily from non-myopic populations.
- *Investigative Approach*: After critical review of the initial findings, the following approach was taken:

1. Discontinuation of the prostaglandin analog to establish true baseline IOP
2. Repeat visual field testing with careful instruction and monitoring, which demonstrated normal findings with good reliability
3. OCT imaging analyzed using the Hood et al. approach of examining the RNFL profile for focal defects rather than relying solely on comparison to normative databases
4. Assessment of the macular ganglion cell complex, which showed symmetrical findings within normal limits without focal defects
5. Stereoscopic disc photographs for baseline documentation of nerve appearance

After comprehensive evaluation, the patient was determined not to have glaucoma but rather typical myopic disc appearance with RNFL distribution patterns common in high myopia. He was scheduled for annual monitoring rather than treatment.

- *Retrospective Analysis*: This case demonstrates several important principles in evaluating myopic patients for glaucoma. As detailed in previous studies (e.g., 69) standard automated parameters on OCT have limited specificity in myopic eyes due to altered distribution of the RNFL and different disc morphology. Their study emphasized that up to 70% of highly myopic eyes without glaucoma may show "abnormal" RNFL measurements when compared to standard normative databases.

The case also illustrates the importance of establishing a solid baseline before initiating treatment. Once initiated, glaucoma therapy often continues indefinitely, making accurate initial diagnosis crucial. The approach of using multiple structural and functional parameters rather than relying on a single technology or measurement better distinguishes physiologic myopic changes from true glaucomatous damage.

Case 10.1.3 The Occult Angle—Missed Angle Closure in Chronic Angle Closure Glaucoma

A 68-year-old female of Middle Eastern descent presented with gradually progressive vision loss and was found to have advanced glaucomatous damage in both eyes. She had been diagnosed with primary open-angle glaucoma five years earlier and was currently using three medications (prostaglandin analog, beta-blocker, and carbonic anhydrase inhibitor) with IOP readings consistently in the low-to-mid 20s mmHg. Her previous records indicated that gonioscopy had been performed at initial diagnosis with notation of "open angles OU."

On examination, visual acuity was 20/30 OD and 20/40 OS. IOPs were 23 mmHg OD and 25 mmHg OS on the three-medication regimen. Anterior chambers appeared quiet but slightly shallow on slit-lamp examination. Gonioscopy revealed appositionally closed angles in both eyes, with peripheral anterior synechiae covering approximately 270 degrees of the angle circumference OU. The remaining visible angle structures showed heavy pigmentation of the trabecular meshwork. Optic nerves demonstrated advanced cupping with C/D ratios of 0.9 OU. Visual fields showed severe constriction with central islands remaining.

- *Diagnostic Challenge*: This case represents a commonly missed diagnosis of chronic angle-closure glaucoma (CACG). The absence of acute symptoms, relatively modest IOP elevation on multiple medications, and initial misclassification led to inappropriate management that failed to address the underlying angle pathology.
- *Investigative Approach*: Based on the gonioscopic findings, the diagnosis was revised to chronic angle-closure glaucoma with extensive synechial closure. The approach included the following:

1. Anterior segment OCT imaging, which confirmed narrow angles with evidence of anterior positioning of the lens
2. Laser peripheral iridotomy performed in both eyes
3. Discontinuation of the prostaglandin analog due to potential exacerbation of inflammation
4. Subsequent laser iridoplasty to further widen the angle in areas without synechiae
5. Cataract extraction with intraocular lens implantation, which significantly deepened the anterior chamber

Following these interventions, IOP decreased to mid-teens on a simplified regimen of a single medication, though the advanced visual field damage remained irreversible.

- *Retrospective Analysis*: This case underscores several critical aspects of angle assessment in glaucoma diagnosis. Gonioscopy remains essential for accurate classification but requires careful technique and interpretation. As highlighted by analyses of angle-closure disease in Middle or Far Eastern populations (70), CACG may present with only modest IOP elevation due to progressive damage to the ciliary body and reduced aqueous production over time. Their study found that up to 25% of presumed POAG cases in their cohort actually had angle closure when subjected to careful gonioscopic and anterior segment imaging assessment.

The case also demonstrates the distinctive management approaches required for different glaucoma mechanisms. While the same IOP-lowering medications are used for both open and closed-angle glaucomas, addressing the underlying angle pathology through iridotomy, iridoplasty, and lens extraction provides more definitive treatment for angle-closure disease.

Case 10.1.4   The Plateau—Recognizing Plateau Iris Configuration

A 42-year-old female presented with elevated IOP of 32 mmHg OD and 28 mmHg OS detected during a routine eye examination. She was asymptomatic with no history of headaches, eye pain, or visual disturbances. Examination revealed clear corneas, deep central anterior chambers, normal-appearing irises without transillumination defects, and open angles on initial gonioscopy. The patient was diagnosed with primary open-angle glaucoma and started on a prostaglandin analog.

Despite good adherence to therapy, follow-up revealed persistently elevated IOPs in the mid-20s mmHg. Additional medications including a beta-blocker and carbonic anhydrase inhibitor provided only modest additional benefit. At a subsequent visit, the patient presented with acute right eye pain, decreased vision, and IOP of 48 mmHg OD with a hazy cornea and shallow peripheral anterior chamber.

- *Diagnostic Challenge*: This case exemplifies the diagnostic difficulty of recognizing plateau iris configuration (PIC) and syndrome (PIS), particularly when central anterior chamber depth appears normal. The initial open-angle appearance on gonioscopy led to misclassification as POAG, while the underlying anatomical predisposition to angle closure went unrecognized.
- *Investigative Approach*: After managing the acute attack with medical therapy, a more detailed evaluation included the following:

1. Careful indentation gonioscopy, which revealed a double-hump sign with anterior insertion of the iris root characteristic of plateau iris configuration
2. Anterior segment OCT showing anteriorly positioned ciliary processes supporting the peripheral iris
3. Ultrasound biomicroscopy confirming the plateau iris configuration with anterior rotation of the ciliary body
4. Laser peripheral iridotomy performed in both eyes
5. Provocative testing with dilation after iridotomy, which demonstrated persistent angle narrowing despite patent iridotomies, confirming plateau iris syndrome

The patient subsequently underwent argon laser peripheral iridoplasty in both eyes, which successfully widened the angle and, in combination with a simplified medication regimen, controlled IOP.

- *Retrospective Analysis*: This case highlights the importance of recognizing anatomical variations that predispose to angle closure even when central anterior chamber depth appears normal. As described by a landmark paper (71) on plateau iris, this condition represents a distinct anatomical configuration that requires specific diagnostic approaches and management strategies different from both typical open-angle and pupillary block angle-closure glaucoma. Their long-term follow-up study demonstrated that plateau iris may account for up to 30% of cases of angle closure in younger patients.

The case also emphasizes the critical role of appropriate gonioscopic technique, including indentation or dynamic gonioscopy, to fully evaluate angle structures and configuration. Simple static gonioscopy may miss subtle findings such as the anterior iris insertion and distinctive "double-hump" sign characteristic of plateau iris. Integration of advanced imaging, particularly ultrasound biomicroscopy which provides visualization of the ciliary body impossible with other techniques, proves especially valuable in these anatomically complex cases.

These challenging diagnostic cases highlight several fundamental principles in glaucoma assessment. First, they underscore the importance of maintaining a broad differential diagnosis, particularly when presentation deviates from typical patterns or response to treatment is suboptimal. Second, they demonstrate the value of comprehensive assessment utilizing multiple complementary diagnostic modalities rather than over-reliance on any single test or finding. Third, they illustrate how recognition of specific patterns and integration of clinical data with an understanding of underlying disease mechanisms can redirect diagnosis and management toward more appropriate and effective approaches. By critically analyzing difficult cases retrospectively, we gain insights that can be applied prospectively to future diagnostic challenges in glaucoma practice.

SECTION 2—UNIQUE SURGICAL CASES AND OUTCOMES

Glaucoma surgery presents some of the most challenging scenarios in ophthalmic practice, requiring careful consideration of anatomical variations, prior interventions, comorbidities, and risk tolerance. Even with meticulous planning and excellent technique, surgical outcomes can be unpredictable, necessitating adaptive approaches and creative problem-solving. This section presents several unique surgical cases that highlight innovative techniques, management of complications, and the critical decision-making processes that drive successful outcomes in complex scenarios.

Case 10.2.1   Management of Failed Trabeculectomy with Conjunctival Scarring

A 62-year-old male with advanced primary open-angle glaucoma presented with uncontrolled intraocular pressure despite maximally tolerated medical therapy. His ocular history included a failed trabeculectomy in the right eye performed three years earlier and a more recent selective laser trabeculoplasty with minimal effect. Examination revealed IOPs of 28 mmHg OD and 24 mmHg OS on four medications. The right eye showed a flat, vascularized bleb with extensive superior conjunctival scarring. Optic nerves demonstrated advanced cupping with C/D ratios of 0.9 OU, and visual fields showed severe constriction with threatened fixation in both eyes.

- *Surgical Challenge*: The case presented multiple challenges: advanced disease requiring substantial pressure reduction, a previously failed filtering procedure, and extensive conjunctival scarring limiting options for conventional filtration surgery. The surgical approach needed to balance efficacy with safety, recognizing the significant risk of vision loss from both surgical complications and continued disease progression.
- *Surgical Approach and Outcome*: After careful consideration of various options, including repeat trabeculectomy with an alternate site, tube shunt implantation, and cyclodestructive procedures, a two-staged approach was planned. First, a Baerveldt glaucoma implant (BGI 350 mm²) was placed in the superotemporal quadrant with tube ligation using a 7–0 polyglactin suture and creation of a venting slit for early pressure control. The tube was positioned in the anterior chamber through a scleral tunnel with patch graft coverage. During the immediate postoperative period, the patient experienced transient hypotony (IOP 4 mmHg) with a shallow anterior chamber, managed conservatively with cycloplegia and activity restriction. By postoperative week six, the chamber had deepened, but IOP had risen to 26 mmHg as the ligature suture effect continued. The planned second stage proceeded with removal of the occluding stent, resulting in immediate IOP reduction to 12 mmHg.

The patient subsequently developed a localized encapsulated bleb around the plate at month three, with IOP rising to 19 mmHg. Bleb needling with subconjunctival mitomycin C was performed in the office, achieving bleb expansion and pressure reduction to 14 mmHg. At one-year follow-up, IOP remained controlled at 15 mmHg on a single medication, with stabilization of visual field defects.

- *Analysis*: This case demonstrates the effective management of a complex scenario where conventional trabeculectomy would likely fail due to conjunctival scarring. The decision to use a large-plate glaucoma drainage device was supported by evidence from the tube versus trabeculectomy (TVT) study, which demonstrated superior success rates for tube shunts compared to trabeculectomy in previously operated eyes (48). The two-stage implantation technique with delayed tube opening helped mitigate early postoperative hypotony, a common complication with large non-valved implants.

The case also highlights the importance of anticipating and managing complications such as encapsulated bleb formation, which occurs in approximately 10–15% of glaucoma drainage device cases. The successful needling procedure illustrates how relatively minor interventions can salvage a partially functioning implant without necessitating complete surgical revision.

Case 10.2.2 Combined Phacoemulsification and Angle-Based MIGS in Pseudoexfoliation Glaucoma

A 74-year-old female with pseudoexfoliation glaucoma presented with progressive visual field deterioration despite IOP in the high teens on three medications. She also had visually significant cataracts reducing acuity to 20/70 OD and 20/50 OS. Examination revealed characteristic pseudoexfoliative material on the anterior lens capsule and pupillary margin, moderately open angles with heavy trabecular pigmentation, and moderate disc cupping with C/D ratios of 0.7 OD and 0.6 OS. The patient reported significant side effects from her glaucoma medications, including ocular surface disease and periorbital fat atrophy from prostaglandin analogs.

- *Surgical Challenge*: This case presented the opportunity to address both cataract and glaucoma simultaneously while potentially reducing medication burden. The primary challenges included increased surgical complexity due to pseudoexfoliation (with potential zonular weakness and small pupil) and selecting the most appropriate MIGS procedure for this specific disease mechanism.
- *Surgical Approach and Outcome*: After discussing various options with the patient, including standalone cataract surgery with continued medical management versus combined approaches with different MIGS procedures, the decision was made to proceed with phacoemulsification combined with gonioscopy-assisted transluminal trabeculotomy (GATT). Surgery began with intracameral epinephrine and placement of a malyugin ring to manage the small pupil. Phacoemulsification proceeded uneventfully with careful hydrodissection and gentle manipulation to avoid zonular stress. A three-piece IOL was placed in the capsular bag. Following IOL implantation, the anterior chamber was deepened with viscoelastic, and a direct gonioscopic view of the nasal angle was obtained. A small goniotomy was created in the trabecular meshwork, and illuminated microcatheter was introduced and advanced 360 degrees through Schlemm's canal. The catheter was then used to perform complete trabeculotomy by gentle traction. The immediate postoperative course was complicated by hyphema, a common occurrence

after GATT, which resolved over two weeks. By postoperative month one, IOP had decreased to 14 mmHg without medications, and visual acuity improved to 20/25. At six-month follow-up, the patient maintained IOP of 16 mmHg on a single medication (from three preoperatively), with resolved ocular surface disease and stabilized visual fields.

- *Analysis*: This case exemplifies the potential benefits of combined cataract extraction and MIGS in appropriate candidates. The selection of GATT rather than other angle-based procedures was influenced by the pathophysiology of pseudoexfoliation glaucoma, which involves deposition of abnormal material and pigment throughout the conventional outflow pathway. As described by studies of GATT outcomes (72, 73) in various glaucoma types, pseudoexfoliation glaucoma responds particularly well to circumferential trabeculotomy, with their series showing mean IOP reduction from 27.3 mmHg to 14.6 mmHg and medication reduction from 3.5 to 1.5 at 12 months. The case also demonstrates important technical considerations for combined surgery in pseudoexfoliation, including strategies for managing small pupils and weak zonules. While the resulting hyphema required additional follow-up, it represented an expected and manageable complication rather than a surgical failure.

Case 10.2.3 Managing Hypotony Maculopathy after Trabeculectomy

A 38-year-old myopic male with juvenile open-angle glaucoma underwent trabeculectomy with mitomycin C in the left eye after inadequate IOP control on maximum medical therapy. The initial postoperative course showed excellent IOP control at 8–10 mmHg with a diffuse, mildly elevated bleb. By postoperative week three, IOP had decreased to 4 mmHg, but the patient remained asymptomatic with visual acuity of 20/20 and normal anterior chamber depth. At the two-month visit, the patient reported new-onset blurred vision with acuity reduced to 20/80. IOP measured 2 mmHg with a diffuse, minimally elevated bleb. Fundus examination revealed chorioretinal folds extending through the macula, and OCT confirmed hypotony maculopathy with retinal striae and choroidal folds.

- *Surgical Challenge*: This case presented the difficult balance between achieving target IOP and avoiding hypotony complications. The management challenge involved resolving hypotony maculopathy while maintaining long-term bleb function and glaucoma control in a young patient with aggressive disease.
- *Surgical Approach and Outcome*: Initial conservative measures included cycloplegia, topical steroid reduction, and large-diameter soft contact lens application, but these failed to resolve the hypotony after three weeks. Surgical intervention was deemed necessary to address the persistent hypotony while attempting to preserve filtering function. Rather than proceeding directly to bleb revision with potential compromise of future filtration, a measured approach was taken using autologous blood injection adjacent to the filtering bleb. Under topical anesthesia, 0.3 mL of autologous blood drawn from the patient was injected subconjunctivally at the posterior margin of the bleb using a 30-gauge needle. The procedure's goal was to induce controlled fibrosis to reduce but not eliminate aqueous filtration. Following the procedure, IOP gradually increased to 6 mmHg at week one, 9 mmHg at week two, and stabilized at 11–12 mmHg by month one. The maculopathy gradually resolved with visual acuity returning to 20/25 by month three. OCT demonstrated resolution of chorioretinal folds, and the patient remained stable with IOP 12–14 mmHg without medications through two years of follow-up.

- *Analysis*: This case highlights the challenge of hypotony management following filtration surgery, particularly in young myopic patients who are at increased risk for this complication. The autologous blood injection technique represents a tissue-sparing approach that allows titrated intervention compared to more invasive bleb revision. A study on the management of post-trabeculectomy hypotony (73) noted success rates of 73–83% with autologous blood injections, though often requiring multiple treatments. They emphasized the importance of intervention before chronic changes develop, as prolonged hypotony can lead to irreversible macular damage.

This case underscores the importance of balancing adequate IOP lowering with the risk of hypotony-related complications. Young age, myopia, and Hispanic ethnicity have all been identified as risk factors for hypotony maculopathy, suggesting that more conservative surgical approaches (including tighter scleral flap sutures, smaller treatment areas for antimetabolites, or consideration of alternative procedures) might be warranted in patients with multiple risk factors.

In summary, these surgical cases illustrate several important principles in the management of complex glaucoma. First, they highlight the value of tailoring surgical approaches to individual patient characteristics, disease mechanisms, and risk factors rather than applying a one-size-fits-all approach. Second, they demonstrate the importance of anticipating potential complications and developing contingency plans before they arise. Third, they underscore the evolving nature of glaucoma surgery, with newer techniques like MIGS offering valuable options for certain patients while traditional approaches remain essential for others. Finally, they reveal how complications, when properly managed, need not represent surgical failures but rather challenges to be overcome through persistent and creative approaches to patient care.

SECTION 3—LESSONS LEARNED FROM COMPLEX CASES

The management of challenging glaucoma cases often yields insights that extend beyond textbook descriptions or clinical trial protocols. These complex scenarios demand integration of theoretical knowledge with practical experience, creative problem-solving, and sometimes departure from standard approaches. This section examines several instructive cases that illustrate broader principles applicable to glaucoma management, highlighting key lessons that can enhance clinical decision-making and patient care.

Case 10.3.1 The Importance of Pressure-Independent Factors in Glaucoma Progression

A 72-year-old female with primary open-angle glaucoma had been followed for 15 years with generally well-controlled intraocular pressure in the low teens. Her treatment regimen included a prostaglandin analog and a combination dorzolamide-timolol preparation. Despite consistently measured IOPs between 12–14 mmHg at office visits, she experienced gradual visual field progression in her left eye over a four-year period, with the mean deviation worsening from −8.4 dB to −14.2 dB.

Comprehensive re-evaluation revealed normal central corneal thickness (545 μm OU), open angles on gonioscopy, and no evidence of secondary glaucoma mechanisms. Review of her medical history identified long-standing systemic hypotension with multiple documented episodes of nocturnal blood pressure drops below 90/60 mmHg. Additionally, she had developed moderate obstructive sleep apnea, diagnosed two years prior but inadequately treated due to CPAP intolerance.

- *Management Approach and Outcome*: Management was modified to address these pressure-independent risk factors. The evening dose of her systemic antihypertensive medication was shifted to morning administration in consultation with her primary care physician. A mandibular advancement device was prescribed as an alternative to CPAP for sleep apnea management. Additionally, the dorzolamide-timolol combination was discontinued given its potential to reduce ocular perfusion through vascular effects, and replaced with brimonidine to maintain IOP control. Following these interventions, ambulatory blood pressure monitoring demonstrated improved nocturnal profiles without compromising daytime control. Sleep studies with the mandibular device showed significant improvement in the apnea-hypopnea index. Visual field testing over the subsequent two years showed stabilization of the mean deviation, with no further progression detected.
- *Lesson Learned*: This case illustrates the critical importance of considering pressure-independent factors in glaucoma management, particularly when progression occurs despite apparently well-controlled IOP. The concept of ocular perfusion pressure (OPP), calculated as the difference between mean arterial pressure and IOP, has emerged as an important consideration in glaucoma management. Multiple population-based studies have identified low OPP as an independent risk factor for glaucoma development and progression. The Barbados eye study found that individuals with lower systolic perfusion pressure had more than twice the risk of developing glaucoma compared to those with normal perfusion pressure (74, 75). Additionally, the case highlights the importance of considering comorbid conditions like obstructive sleep apnea, which has been independently associated with glaucoma in multiple studies. While measuring IOP remains the cornerstone of glaucoma assessment, identifying and addressing pressure-independent risk factors can significantly impact long-term outcomes, particularly in patients demonstrating progression despite seemingly adequate pressure control.

Case 10.3.2   Recognizing Steroid-Induced Glaucoma in Complex Medical Scenarios

A 56-year-old male with moderate primary open-angle glaucoma and well-controlled IOP on bimatoprost monotherapy experienced an acute anterior uveitis in his right eye. Initial management included frequent topical prednisolone acetate 1% and cyclopentolate 1% for comfort and prevention of synechiae. After two weeks of treatment, his anterior chamber inflammation had significantly improved, but IOP had increased from a baseline of 16 mmHg to 32 mmHg. Additional topical medications (dorzolamide-timolol combination and brimonidine) were added, and topical steroid was tapered, achieving modest IOP reduction to 26 mmHg.

Three weeks later, despite further steroid tapering and continued maximum topical therapy, IOP remained elevated at 28 mmHg. Careful anterior segment examination revealed white crystalline deposits on the anterior lens surface and trabecular meshwork visible on gonioscopy. Upon detailed questioning, the patient disclosed that he had been receiving triamcinolone injections from his rheumatologist for shoulder pain, with the most recent injection administered two days before his uveitis presentation. Additionally, he had been using a prescribed dermatologic cream containing clobetasol for facial rash.

- *Management Approach and Outcome*: Recognition of the steroid-induced component led to a multidimensional approach. Communication with the patient's rheumatologist resulted in transitioning from triamcinolone to a non-steroidal alternative for his shoulder condition. The dermatologist substituted the clobetasol with tacrolimus ointment. For the ocular inflammation, prednisolone was replaced with loteprednol, a soft steroid with less impact on IOP.

Despite these measures, IOP remained elevated at 24 mmHg after two additional weeks. Selective laser trabeculoplasty was performed, yielding modest initial benefit. Ultimately, the patient required a trabeculectomy with mitomycin C, which successfully controlled IOP at 12 mmHg with concurrent resolution of inflammation.

- *Lesson Learned*: This case underscores the importance of recognizing steroid-induced glaucoma in patients with complex medical profiles and multiple potential sources of steroid exposure. Beyond topical ocular steroids, clinicians must consider injectable, inhaled, dermatologic, and oral sources, which can contribute to ocular hypertension through various mechanisms. The classic appearance of crystalline deposits on the anterior lens surface ("steroid-induced cataract") served as an important diagnostic clue in this case. The case also highlights the concept of steroid responsiveness, which exists along a continuum rather than as a binary characteristic. Approximately 5% of the population demonstrates high steroid responsiveness with significant IOP elevation after minimal exposure, while another 35% shows intermediate responsiveness. Individuals with pre-existing POAG have a substantially higher risk of steroid response, with studies suggesting rates of 60–90% depending on steroid potency and duration of exposure.

Management strategies include identifying and eliminating unnecessary steroid exposures, substituting lower-potency alternatives when steroids are required, considering non-steroidal alternatives for inflammatory conditions, and implementing appropriate IOP-lowering therapies. In cases with severe or refractory IOP elevation, surgical intervention may become necessary despite addressing the underlying steroid trigger.

Case 10.3.3 The Challenge of Medication Non-Adherence in Glaucoma Management

A 68-year-old female with advanced primary open-angle glaucoma demonstrated progressive visual field loss despite an apparently optimal medical regimen including a prostaglandin analog, brimonidine, and dorzolamide-timolol fixed combination. Office-measured IOPs consistently ranged from 18–22 mmHg, higher than the target pressure of 15 mmHg established based on her disease severity. The patient repeatedly affirmed perfect medication adherence during clinic visits. Given the progressive field loss and suboptimal IOP control, trabeculectomy was recommended and scheduled. During the preoperative evaluation, a comprehensive medication reconciliation revealed she was taking 14 different systemic medications for various chronic conditions. When asked to demonstrate her eye drop technique, she exhibited multiple errors including missing the eye, instilling multiple drops, and failing to close the puncta. Further discussion revealed significant confusion about her medication schedule and difficulty remembering doses due to cognitive changes she had not previously disclosed.

- *Management Approach and Outcome*: Rather than proceeding directly to surgery, a medication simplification approach was implemented. Her three topical medications were replaced with a fixed-combination of latanoprostene bunod and netarsudil administered once daily. Her daughter was engaged to assist with medication administration and electronic medication reminders were implemented. The patient was provided with a punctal occlusion device to improve topical drug delivery. Three months later, IOP had decreased to 14–16 mmHg on the simplified regimen with documented adherence. Visual field testing showed stabilization of previously progressive defects. The scheduled trabeculectomy was postponed in favor of continued monitoring with the successful medical regimen.
- *Lesson Learned*: This case highlights the critical importance of identifying and addressing medication non-adherence before concluding medical therapy failure and proceeding to surgical intervention. Studies consistently demonstrate that adherence to glaucoma medications is poor, with objective monitoring showing rates of approximately 50–60% in many patient populations. The Glaucoma Adherence and Persistency Study (GAPS) revealed multiple factors associated with poor adherence, including complex dosing regimens, side effects, cost concerns, and inadequate understanding of the disease (43). The case also demonstrates the value of direct observation of medication administration technique, comprehensive medication reconciliation, and assessment of potential barriers to adherence including cognitive function, physical limitations, and health literacy. Simplifying medication regimens, utilizing fixed-combination preparations, involving family members in care, and implementing reminder systems represent evidence-based approaches to improving adherence. In some cases, these interventions may achieve target pressure control without requiring surgical intervention, though the decision to postpone surgery must be accompanied by vigilant monitoring for continued disease stability.

Concluding the section, these complex cases illustrate several overarching principles essential to effective glaucoma management. First, they demonstrate the importance of looking beyond intraocular pressure alone to consider the multifactorial nature of glaucoma progression, including vascular factors, medication effects, and adherence challenges. Second, they highlight the value of thorough history-taking, including medication reconciliation across all healthcare providers and administration routes. Third, they underscore the significance of direct observation and practical assessment of patient capabilities rather than relying solely on self-reporting.

Perhaps most importantly, these cases reveal the iterative nature of glaucoma management, where treatment plans require continual reassessment and modification based on clinical response and emerging information. By maintaining a comprehensive perspective that integrates ocular findings with systemic considerations, medication effects, and practical patient factors, clinicians can develop more effective individualized approaches to challenging glaucoma cases.

CHAPTER 11
LIVING WITH
GLAUCOMA

While previous chapters have addressed the scientific and clinical aspects of glaucoma, this chapter turns our attention to the profound human experience of living with the disease. Glaucoma affects not merely the eyes but the whole person—their daily functioning, emotional well-being, social relationships, and sense of identity. For many patients, the diagnosis marks the beginning of a lifelong journey that demands adaptation, resilience, and support. Understanding this lived experience is essential for clinicians seeking to provide truly comprehensive care that addresses both the physiological and psychological dimensions of the disease.

The impact of glaucoma extends far beyond the clinical metrics of intraocular pressure, visual field indices, and medication regimens that typically dominate professional discourse. Patients navigate complex practical challenges including medication management, financial burdens, transportation difficulties, occupational limitations, and the fear of progressive vision loss. Simultaneously, they contend with less visible burdens: anxiety about the future, grief over actual or anticipated losses, strained relationships, and the cognitive effort of adapting to changing visual abilities. These experiences unfold against the backdrop of a condition that remains largely invisible to others, creating a disconnect between patients' internal experience and external perceptions.

This chapter explores the realities of living with glaucoma through three complementary perspectives. First, we present authentic patient narratives that illuminate the diverse ways individuals experience and make meaning of their diagnosis. These stories reveal both common themes and unique circumstances that shape each person's journey. Second, we examine evidence-based strategies for coping with the psychological challenges of glaucoma, recognizing that emotional well-being significantly influences both quality of life and treatment adherence. Finally, we consider how advocacy and support systems can empower patients, reduce isolation, and transform the individual experience of glaucoma into collective action that benefits the broader community.

By centering the lived experience of glaucoma, this chapter aims to foster greater empathy and understanding among healthcare providers while offering practical insights for supporting patients beyond clinical interventions. It recognizes that optimal glaucoma management involves not only preserving vision but also maintaining quality of life, fostering psychological resilience, and honoring the expertise that patients develop through living with their condition each day.

DOI: 10.1201/9781003646693-11

SECTION I—PATIENT STORIES AND TESTIMONIALS

Patient narratives provide a window into the lived experience of glaucoma that clinical descriptions alone cannot capture. These first-person accounts reveal the diverse ways individuals interpret, respond to, and integrate their diagnosis into their lives. By listening to these stories, clinicians gain valuable insights that can inform more empathetic and effective care. This section presents several patient testimonials that highlight common themes in the glaucoma journey while acknowledging the unique circumstances that shape each individual's experience.

Diagnosis and Early Adjustment: Ms. E's Story

"I was 42 when my doctor noticed something concerning during a routine eye exam and referred me to a specialist. I remember sitting in the examination room while the ophthalmologist explained that I had primary open-angle glaucoma. He used terms like 'intraocular pressure' and 'optic nerve damage,' but all I could think was: 'Am I going blind?' I had no symptoms—my vision seemed perfect—so the diagnosis felt completely abstract, like it was happening to someone else. The first year was the hardest. Learning to use eye drops correctly took weeks of practice. I'd miss my eye, waste drops, or flinch and blink them out. Nobody warned me about the burning sensation or that some drops would make my eyes red. I hid my diagnosis from colleagues at first, embarrassed when I had to excuse myself to put in my afternoon dose.

"What surprised me most was the emotional impact. I found myself grieving for a future loss that hadn't happened yet. I'd look at my children's faces and wonder if one day I wouldn't be able to see them clearly. These thoughts would ambush me at random moments—while driving, during work meetings, or when reading bedtime stories to my kids. Six years later, my glaucoma is stable, and those early fears have subsided. I've learned to incorporate my medication routine into daily life until it became almost automatic. The regular check-ups still cause anxiety—I find myself holding my breath when the doctor examines my visual field results—but I've accepted that glaucoma is now part of my life story, not its defining feature."

Ms. E's account illustrates the common disconnect many patients experience between an asymptomatic condition and its serious implications. Her story highlights the practical challenges of treatment adherence and the emotional work of integrating a chronic disease into one's identity. The gradual transition from acute distress to acceptance represents a typical psychological adjustment pattern observed in many chronic conditions.

Progressive Vision Loss: Mr. R's Journey

"I was diagnosed with glaucoma in my late fifties, though my doctors suspect I'd had it for years before it was caught. By then, I'd already lost significant peripheral vision in my right eye. I initially thought the medications would fix everything, but my doctor explained that the damage was permanent—we could only try to prevent further loss. The progression was so gradual that I adapted without fully realizing how much my vision had changed. I'd bump into door frames occasionally or miss objects on my right side, but I'd attribute it to clumsiness or distraction. It wasn't until I failed a driving test renewal that I had to confront how significantly my visual field had narrowed. Giving up driving was the first major lifestyle change that made my condition real. My wife became my chauffeur, and I felt my independence slipping away. Simple errands now required planning and coordination. I retired earlier than planned from my accounting practice when I could no longer reliably read financial statements. The hardest adjustment has been social. I've stopped attending large gatherings because I can't navigate crowded rooms comfortably or recognize faces until people are directly in front of me. Friends stopped inviting us to dinner parties after I knocked over a wine glass reaching for bread I couldn't see properly. My world has gradually contracted. What's helped most is connecting with others who understand. In my support group, I don't have to explain myself when I miss a handshake or walk hesitantly in a new environment. I've learned practical adaptations from others further along in their glaucoma journey—high-contrast tape on stair edges, lighting strategies, organizational systems for medications. Most importantly, I've learned that there's life after vision loss, even if it's a different life than I'd planned."

Mr. R's testimonial captures the functional and social consequences of progressive vision loss. His experience reflects findings from qualitative research on the psychosocial impact of glaucoma. A study (76) documented how visual field loss affects daily activities and social participation, with participants reporting increased dependency, activity limitation, and social isolation similar to Robert's experience. His account also highlights the value of peer support in providing both practical strategies and psychological validation.

Young-Onset Experience: Ms. M's Perspective

"Being diagnosed with glaucoma at 26 set me apart from both my peers and typical glaucoma patients. When I mention my condition, people often say, 'But that's an old person's disease!' This misconception makes it harder to find understanding among friends my age who can't relate to managing a chronic condition or worrying about future vision loss when they're focused on careers and relationships. The treatment burden feels particularly heavy at this stage of life. Remembering eye drops while traveling for work or staying over with friends requires planning. Dating comes with the awkward moment of explaining why I have medication in my purse and alarms set on my phone. I worry about how potential partners will react to the possibility of worsening vision in our future. Financial concerns are also significant. I've chosen jobs based on health insurance coverage rather than career advancement. The co-pays for medications, specialist appointments, and procedures add up, affecting my ability to save for major life milestones like home ownership. Looking ahead, I worry about having children—both the genetic implications and whether my vision will limit my ability to parent as actively as I'd like.

"What helps me cope is reframing my early diagnosis as an advantage. Because we caught it young, I've been able to preserve most of my vision. I've become an advocate, raising awareness about glaucoma screening for younger adults. I'm methodical about my treatment regimen, using tech solutions like medication tracking apps. And I've learned to be open about my condition, which has actually strengthened some relationships and weeded out people who can't handle health challenges."

Ms. M's story highlights the unique challenges of managing glaucoma during young adulthood, a period typically associated with independence and future planning rather than health limitations. Her narrative reflects research on the psychological burden of early-onset chronic disease, including identity disruption, financial strain, and concerns about life transitions. Her experience also demonstrates the potential for post-traumatic growth, wherein individuals derive meaning and purpose from adversity through advocacy and helping others.

Cultural Perspectives: Mr. A's Experience

"In my community, eye diseases aren't discussed openly. When I was diagnosed with glaucoma at 65, my first instinct was to keep it private. Among my extended family and church members, there's a perspective that health problems, especially those affecting vision, are simply part of aging—something to be endured rather than treated aggressively. This cultural context affected my early approach to treatment. When my doctor prescribed daily eye drops, I used them sporadically, particularly when symptoms like mild eye pain or headaches occurred. I didn't understand that the medication was preventative rather than symptomatic. My doctor seemed frustrated with my 'non-compliance,' but I never explained my reasoning or the influence of my community's health beliefs. A turning point came when my family member, himself diagnosed with glaucoma, spoke openly during a family meeting about the importance of treatment. His standing in our family gave permission for others to share their experiences. I discovered that several respected elders were successfully managing the same condition. Now I approach my glaucoma management differently. I've become more comfortable asking questions during appointments and expressing concerns about medication side effects or costs. I organize monthly health discussions at our community center where eye specialists speak about common conditions affecting our neighborhood. And I've worked with my doctor to find a treatment schedule that accommodates my daily routine, making adherence much easier."

Mr. A's testimonial illustrates how cultural contexts and community norms influence health behaviors and treatment engagement. Research on cultural factors affecting glaucoma care has documented substantial variations in disease conceptualization, stigma, and treatment expectations across different communities (77). James's experience demonstrates how culturally sensitive interventions—particularly those involving respected community members—can bridge the gap between clinical recommendations and patient implementation.

All these patient narratives presented in the previous section, while representing individual experiences, reveal several common themes in living with glaucoma. The emotional journey from diagnosis through adjustment involves navigating uncertainty, grief, and eventually finding ways to integrate the condition into one's identity. Practical challenges include treatment management, financial considerations, and adapting to functional limitations. Social dimensions encompass disclosure decisions, changing relationship dynamics, and accessing supportive communities.

By centralizing these lived experiences, healthcare providers gain a more complete understanding of glaucoma beyond its clinical parameters. Effective care must address not only the physiological aspects of the disease but also its psychological, social, and practical impacts on patients' lives. These narratives also demonstrate the resilience and adaptability of individuals living with glaucoma, who often develop expertise in managing their condition that complements professional knowledge in meaningful ways.

SECTION 2—COPING STRATEGIES AND MENTAL HEALTH

The psychological impact of glaucoma extends far beyond the clinical management of intraocular pressure and visual field preservation. Living with a chronic, potentially blinding eye disease presents significant mental health challenges that can affect quality of life, treatment adherence, and ultimately, clinical outcomes. This section examines the psychological dimensions of glaucoma and evidence-based strategies to support patients' mental well-being throughout their disease journey.

Receiving a glaucoma diagnosis initiates a complex psychological adjustment process for many patients. Initial reactions often include shock, disbelief, anxiety, and fear of blindness. These responses may occur even in patients with early-stage disease and minimal visual impairment, as the diagnosis introduces uncertainty about future vision and functioning. As patients transition from acute adjustment to long-term management, different psychological challenges emerge at various stages of the disease. Anxiety and depression occur at significantly higher rates among glaucoma patients compared to the general population. In a previous study it was found that the prevalence of depression in glaucoma patients ranged from 10.9% to 32.1%, substantially higher than age-matched controls (78). Anxiety rates showed similar elevation, with particular peaks during diagnosis, after disease progression, and when initiating new treatments or considering surgical interventions.

Several factors contribute to this increased psychological burden. Fear of blindness represents a universal concern, particularly given glaucoma's progressive nature. Treatment-related anxiety includes worry about medication side effects, surgical complications, and the financial burden of ongoing care. For patients experiencing vision loss, anxiety often centers on maintaining independence, employment, and social connections. Depression may manifest as sadness, loss of interest in previously enjoyed activities, sleep disturbances, or feelings of hopelessness about the future. In some patients, depression emerges directly from vision loss and associated functional limitations. In others, it relates to the chronic stress of disease management, social isolation, or diminished self-efficacy. Importantly, depression can create a negative feedback loop by reducing motivation for treatment adherence, appointment attendance, and engagement in vision rehabilitation.

Glaucoma's unpredictable course creates persistent uncertainty that many patients find particularly challenging. Despite optimal treatment, some patients experience continued progression while others remain stable for years. This unpredictability can undermine patients' sense of control and complicate long-term life planning. Many report difficulty balancing reasonable preparation for potential vision loss with maintaining optimism and present-focused living.

The invisible nature of early glaucoma further complicates psychological adjustment. Patients often appear entirely well to others despite experiencing significant anxiety about their condition and its management. This invisibility can lead to decreased social support and understanding from family members, employers, and even healthcare providers who may underestimate the psychological burden of an asymptomatic condition.

Research on psychological interventions for glaucoma patients remains limited compared to other chronic conditions. However, several approaches have demonstrated effectiveness in supporting mental well-being while enhancing disease management and quality of life.

Knowledge plays a critical role in psychological adaptation to chronic illness. Patients who understand their condition, treatment options, and prognosis generally demonstrate better psychological adjustment than those with limited or inaccurate information. However, information needs vary substantially between individuals. Some patients seek comprehensive knowledge about their disease, while others prefer focused information directly relevant to their current situation. Effective patient education includes several key components: clear explanation of diagnosis using accessible language, visual aids demonstrating disease mechanisms, realistic discussion of prognosis that balances honesty with hope, practical instruction in treatment administration, and appropriate pacing of information to prevent overwhelm. Written materials and reputable online resources provide reinforcement of verbal education and allow patients to review information at their own pace.

The timing of educational interventions also influences their effectiveness. At diagnosis, patients often benefit from focused information addressing immediate concerns and treatment requirements, with more comprehensive education introduced gradually as they adjust emotionally. During disease progression or treatment changes, targeted education addressing specific new challenges helps restore a sense of control and competence.

Practical coping strategies that enhance patients' sense of control over daily challenges show particular promise in improving quality of life with glaucoma. These approaches include:

- *Medication management techniques to overcome common adherence barriers.* Simplified dosing regimens, medication organizers, electronic reminders, and integration of eye drop administration into existing daily routines can reduce treatment burden. For patients with dexterity issues or difficulty with self-administration, adaptive devices and family member training may prove beneficial.
- *Environmental modifications to accommodate changing visual needs.* Strategies include enhanced lighting without glare, high-contrast visual cues; organizational systems for personal items, and home safety adaptations to

prevent falls. Introducing these modifications gradually helps patients maintain independence while acknowledging changing abilities.

- *Practical problem-solving for specific functional challenges.* This approach involves identifying problematic situations (such as reading menus in dimly lit restaurants or recognizing faces in social settings), brainstorming potential solutions, evaluating options, implementing the most promising strategy, and assessing its effectiveness. This structured process builds resilience and adaptability while reinforcing patients' problem-solving capacity.
- *Communicating effectively about vision limitations.* Many patients benefit from developing clear, concise explanations of their condition for different audiences (family, friends, colleagues, strangers) and practicing direct requests for needed accommodations. This approach reduces social awkwardness while ensuring appropriate support.

Cognitive-behavioral techniques address the interconnection between thoughts, emotions, and behaviors, helping patients develop more adaptive patterns in each domain. These approaches have demonstrated effectiveness across numerous chronic conditions and show promise specifically for glaucoma patients.

- *Cognitive restructuring* helps patients identify and modify unhelpful thought patterns that contribute to distress. Common examples include catastrophizing about potential blindness, all-or-nothing thinking about visual abilities, or excessive self-blame for disease progression. By examining evidence for and against these thoughts and developing more balanced perspectives, patients can reduce anxiety and depression while maintaining realistic hope.
- *Acceptance-based strategies* focus on acknowledging current realities while committing to valued activities despite challenges. Rather than fighting against unchangeable aspects of their condition, patients learn to direct energy toward meaningful engagement within existing limitations. This approach proves particularly valuable for addressing the uncertainty inherent in glaucoma.
- *Mindfulness practices* cultivate present-moment awareness without judgment, helping patients manage anxiety about future vision loss. Brief mindfulness exercises can be integrated into daily routines, including during drop administration or doctor's appointments, creating opportunities to reduce stress throughout the disease management process.
- *Social support* significantly influences psychological adjustment to chronic illness. For glaucoma patients, meaningful connection with others who understand their experience can reduce isolation and normalize emotional responses. Structured support groups provide both informational and emotional benefits through shared problem-solving and mutual understanding. Online communities offer accessible options for patients with transportation limitations or those preferring anonymity. Beyond peer support, maintaining and strengthening existing social connections helps prevent the isolation that often accompanies progressive vision impairment. Proactive communication with family members about specific support needs—whether practical assistance or emotional validation—enhances relationship quality while reducing caregiver burden and patient dependence.

While many patients manage the psychological aspects of glaucoma through the strategies described previously, some benefit from professional mental health intervention. Indicators for referral include persistent depression or anxiety symptoms, significant functional impairment due to psychological distress, suicidal ideation, substance use as a coping mechanism, or inadequate social support systems.

Several therapeutic approaches show particular promise for glaucoma patients. Individual cognitive-behavioral therapy addresses specific anxiety and depression symptoms while building coping skills. Acceptance and commitment therapy (ACT) helps patients live meaningfully despite uncertainty and potential loss. Family therapy supports adjustment of the entire household system to the challenges of chronic eye disease. Psychotropic medications may be appropriate adjuncts for patients with moderate to severe depression or anxiety, ideally prescribed in collaboration between psychiatric providers and ophthalmologists to monitor potential interactions with glaucoma medications or effects on intraocular pressure.

Addressing the psychological aspects of glaucoma need not require extensive additional resources within busy clinical settings. Simple practices that can be integrated into routine care include the following: screening for psychological distress using brief validated measures or targeted questions about mood, anxiety, and coping during regular appointments; creating space for patients to express concerns by asking open-ended questions about their experience of living with glaucoma, beyond symptom reports; normalizing emotional responses by acknowledging that anxiety and mood changes are common in chronic eye disease; maintaining a balanced approach that addresses both biomedical and psychosocial aspects of the condition during clinical encounters; and developing referral relationships with mental health professionals interested in chronic illness adjustment.

A comprehensive approach to glaucoma management recognizes that psychological well-being and disease outcomes are inextricably linked through multiple pathways. By supporting patients' psychological adaptation and coping skills, clinicians not only improve quality of life but potentially enhance treatment adherence, appointment attendance, and active participation in disease management—all factors that ultimately influence long-term visual outcomes.

SECTION 3—A VISION FOR ADVOCACY AND SUPPORT

Beyond clinical management and individual coping strategies, collective advocacy and structured support systems play vital roles in improving the lives of people with glaucoma. These efforts transform isolated personal challenges into opportunities for systemic change, community building, and knowledge advancement. This section explores how advocacy initiatives, support networks, and collaborative approaches can enhance the glaucoma journey while contributing to broader progress in prevention, treatment, and public awareness.

Patient advocacy in glaucoma operates across multiple levels, from individual self-advocacy in clinical encounters to organized efforts influencing policy and research priorities. At its core, advocacy represents the process of actively participating in decisions affecting one's health and well-being while working to improve conditions for others with similar experiences. Effective self-advocacy begins with patients developing the knowledge, confidence, and communication skills to participate actively in their healthcare. This includes preparing questions before appointments, requesting clarification of unfamiliar terms, expressing concerns about treatment side effects or costs, and participating meaningfully in treatment decisions. For many patients, becoming an effective self-advocate requires overcoming traditional power dynamics in healthcare relationships and recognizing their own expertise about living with their condition.

Healthcare providers can support patient self-advocacy by creating environments that welcome questions, providing adequate time for discussion, respecting patient preferences, and explicitly inviting partnership in decision-making. This collaborative approach not only improves patient satisfaction but often leads to treatment plans better aligned with individuals' values and circumstances, potentially enhancing adherence and outcomes.

Beyond individual healthcare interactions, collective advocacy efforts address broader systemic issues affecting the glaucoma community. Patient organizations like the Glaucoma Research Foundation and the International Glaucoma Association have successfully advocated for increased research funding, improved access to care, enhanced insurance coverage for treatments, and greater public awareness of the disease. These organizations amplify patient voices through multiple channels: gathering and presenting patient perspectives to regulatory agencies reviewing new treatments, providing testimony for legislative hearings on healthcare policy, participating in research priority-setting processes, and developing relationships with industry partners to ensure patient needs inform product development. The most effective advocacy organizations integrate diverse patient experiences, including those from underrepresented populations who often face additional barriers to glaucoma care. By centering equity in their work, these groups help address disparities in glaucoma diagnosis, treatment access, and outcomes that disproportionately affect certain racial, ethnic, geographic, and socioeconomic groups.

Support networks provide essential emotional connection, practical assistance, and information exchange for people with glaucoma. These networks take various forms, each offering unique benefits while serving complementary functions in a comprehensive support ecosystem. Professionally facilitated support groups provide safe spaces for glaucoma patients to share experiences, exchange coping strategies, and receive emotional validation. These groups may be organized through eye care institutions, community organizations, or patient advocacy groups, with formats ranging from time-limited educational series to ongoing open forums. Some target specific populations, such as newly diagnosed patients, those with advanced vision loss, or family caregivers.

Research demonstrates multiple benefits from participation in structured support groups. Members report decreased feelings of isolation, improved disease knowledge, enhanced coping skills, and greater confidence in communicating with healthcare providers. For some participants, these groups also serve as gateways to involvement in broader advocacy efforts, transforming personal challenges into motivation for systemic change.

One-to-one peer support offers a valuable alternative or complement to group settings. In these programs, experienced glaucoma patients provide individualized guidance to those newly diagnosed or facing significant transitions like surgery or advancing vision loss. The shared lived experience creates a foundation of understanding that differs from professional support, while the personalized format allows for focused attention on specific concerns. Effective peer mentoring programs include careful matching of mentors and mentees, thorough training for mentors, clear boundaries regarding medical advice, and professional oversight. When well-implemented, these programs demonstrate high satisfaction among both mentors, who find meaning in helping others navigate familiar challenges, and mentees, who benefit from practical wisdom and emotional reassurance.

Digital platforms have revolutionized support options for glaucoma patients, particularly those with mobility limitations, geographic isolation, or preferences for anonymity. Online forums, social media groups, and virtual meetups provide continuous access to peer wisdom and emotional support independent of location or time constraints. These communities prove especially valuable for patients with rare glaucoma subtypes or unusual circumstances who might never encounter similar individuals in local settings.

Beyond convenience, online communities offer unique benefits: searchable archives of previous discussions, opportunities to learn from patients across different healthcare systems and treatment approaches, and the ability to process information at one's own pace. However, they also present challenges, including potential misinformation, lack of professional oversight, and limited ability to verify credentials or experiences of participants. The most effective support and advocacy approaches integrate multiple stakeholders—patients, healthcare providers, researchers, industry representatives, and policymakers—in collaborative efforts toward shared goals. Several models demonstrate particular promise.

Increasingly, research funders and institutions recognize the value of meaningful patient involvement throughout the research process. Patient-centered research initiatives involve glaucoma patients as partners rather than merely subjects, from establishing research priorities to designing studies, interpreting results, and disseminating findings. This approach ensures that research addresses questions most relevant to patients' lived experiences and produces outcomes that meaningfully improve quality of life.

The Patient-Centered Outcomes Research Institute (PCORI) has supported several significant glaucoma studies employing this collaborative methodology. These projects typically examine questions about treatment burden, quality of life impact, and practical management challenges that traditionally received less attention than biological mechanisms or pressure-lowering efficacy but hold critical importance for patients navigating daily life with glaucoma.

Integrated Care Networks

Comprehensive glaucoma management extends beyond ophthalmological care to encompass psychological support, visual rehabilitation, community services, and practical assistance. Integrated care networks coordinate these varied resources, creating seamless pathways for patients to access appropriate support at each stage of their journey. In well-developed integrated models, ophthalmologists collaborate closely with optometrists, low vision specialists, mental health professionals, social workers, and community organizations. Electronic referral systems, shared documentation, and regular interdisciplinary communication ensure continuity of care without requiring patients to navigate complex systems independently during periods of vision or emotional distress.

Technological innovations increasingly enhance both clinical care and supportive services for glaucoma patients. Telehealth platforms extend specialist access to underserved areas, smartphone applications support medication adherence through automated reminders and tracking, and assistive technologies help maintain independence despite vision changes. Patient communities provide valuable feedback on these tools, ensuring they address actual rather than presumed needs.

A comprehensive vision for glaucoma advocacy and support recognizes the interconnection between individual experiences and systemic conditions, between clinical care and community resources, and between current needs and future possibilities. By fostering robust advocacy initiatives and multilayered support networks, the glaucoma community transforms individual challenges into collective progress. Healthcare providers play essential roles in this ecosystem—not only by providing expert clinical care but also by connecting patients to appropriate resources, supporting self-advocacy, and participating in collaborative efforts to improve the overall landscape of glaucoma care and support.

CHAPTER 12
CONCLUSION

The Road Ahead—A Call to Action for Researchers, Clinicians, and Policymakers

The journey of understanding and managing glaucoma represents one of the most complex and compelling challenges in modern medical science. As we stand at the intersection of remarkable scientific progress and persistent global health challenges, the path forward demands a fundamental reimagining of our approach to this sight-threatening disease. The landscape of glaucoma care is defined by both extraordinary achievements and profound limitations—a narrative of scientific brilliance tempered by the sobering reality of millions living with undiagnosed or inadequately managed vision loss.

The global burden of glaucoma presents a stark mathematical and humanitarian challenge. With approximately 80 million people affected worldwide, and projections suggesting this number will exceed 111 million by 2040, we are confronting a public health crisis of significant magnitude. Perhaps most alarming is the fact that up to 90% of cases remain undiagnosed in various populations, representing a massive gap between scientific knowledge and practical implementation. This disconnect is not merely a statistical anomaly but a profound human tragedy, with each undetected case representing a potential lifetime of preventable vision loss.

The complexity of glaucoma extends far beyond simple numeric representations. It is a disease that intersects with nearly every aspect of human health and experience. Genetic predispositions, environmental factors, systemic health conditions, and socioeconomic circumstances all play crucial roles in its development, progression, and impact. This multidimensional nature demands an equally sophisticated and holistic approach to research, prevention, and treatment. For researchers, the road ahead demands a radical reimagining of scientific inquiry. The traditional reductionist approach that focuses narrowly on intraocular pressure must give way to a more holistic, interdisciplinary understanding of glaucoma. We must embrace a precision medicine paradigm that integrates genetic, molecular, environmental, and clinical data to develop truly personalized risk assessment and treatment strategies. This requires breaking down traditional disciplinary silos and creating collaborative research ecosystems that can tackle the disease's complex pathophysiology from multiple angles.

The scientific community must also expand its conceptual frameworks. Glaucoma can no longer be viewed simply as an eye disease, but as a complex neurodegenerative

DOI: 10.1201/9781003646693-12

condition with profound implications for patients' overall health and quality of life. Research must explore the web of connections between glaucoma and broader neurological, vascular, and systemic health processes. This expanded perspective opens new avenues for understanding disease mechanisms, developing innovative treatments, and potentially preventing vision loss before it begins.

The clinical landscape must simultaneously undergo a profound transformation. Healthcare providers can no longer view glaucoma as a purely ophthalmological condition to be managed through periodic pressure measurements and medication adjustments. Instead, a comprehensive, patient-centered approach is essential—one that addresses the psychological, social, and functional dimensions of living with a progressive eye disease. This means integrating mental health support, rehabilitation strategies, and patient education into standard care protocols, recognizing that effective management extends far beyond clinical metrics.

Technological innovation offers unprecedented opportunities to revolutionize glaucoma care. Artificial intelligence, advanced imaging technologies, genetic profiling, and emerging diagnostic tools are not simply incremental improvements but potential paradigm-shifting approaches. These technologies promise a future where glaucoma might be detected before irreversible damage occurs, where progression can be precisely monitored and potentially halted, and where personalized interventions can be tailored to individual risk profiles with unprecedented accuracy.

The transformative potential of technology extends beyond diagnostic capabilities. Emerging therapeutic approaches, including gene therapies, stem cell treatments, and novel drug delivery systems, offer glimpses of a future where vision loss might be prevented or even reversed. The convergence of computational biology, molecular medicine, and advanced imaging technologies creates an ecosystem of innovation that could fundamentally reshape our understanding and treatment of glaucoma.

Policymakers play a critical role in this transformative journey. Healthcare systems must be redesigned to prioritize preventive eye care, with mandatory comprehensive eye examinations for high-risk populations, expanded insurance coverage for screening and treatment, and integrated care models that connect ophthalmological services with primary healthcare. This requires a fundamental shift from reactive to proactive healthcare strategies, recognizing that investment in early detection and management produces substantial long-term economic and humanitarian benefits.

The challenge of health equity must be at the forefront of our collective efforts. Glaucoma disproportionately affects vulnerable populations, with significant disparities in diagnosis, treatment, and outcomes across racial, ethnic, and socioeconomic groups. Addressing these disparities requires more than well-intentioned interventions—it demands a committed, systemic approach that acknowledges and actively works to dismantle the structural barriers that prevent equitable access to eye care.

The cultural dimensions of glaucoma management cannot be overlooked. Healthcare approaches must become increasingly sophisticated in their cultural competence, recognizing that disease understanding, treatment adherence, and healthcare-seeking behaviors are profoundly influenced by cultural contexts. This requires developing communication strategies, educational materials, and care models that respect and integrate diverse health beliefs and practices.

International collaboration emerges as a critical imperative. The global nature of glaucoma demands coordinated efforts that transcend national boundaries. Research institutions, healthcare providers, technology companies, and policymakers must create robust networks that can share knowledge, resources, and innovative approaches. This collaborative ecosystem should prioritize knowledge transfer, particularly supporting research and healthcare development in resource-limited settings.

The psychological and social dimensions of glaucoma represent an often-overlooked frontier of medical research and care. Beyond the physiological management of the disease, we must develop comprehensive support systems that address the emotional challenges of living with a progressive eye condition. This includes developing robust mental health support mechanisms, peer support networks, and rehabilitation strategies that empower patients to maintain quality of life and psychological resilience.

As we look to the future, hope and determination must be our guiding principles. The road ahead is complex, challenging, and uncertain, but not insurmountable. By approaching glaucoma with scientific rigor, clinical compassion, and an unwavering commitment to global health equity, we can transform this silent threat into a manageable, and potentially preventable, condition.

Our collective goal transcends scientific achievement—it is fundamentally about preserving human potential. Each advancement, each breakthrough, each moment of compassionate care represents a commitment to ensuring that no individual loses their vision to a preventable or treatable disease. The journey continues, and every step matters.

REFERENCES

1. Leffler CT, Schwartz SG, Hadi TM, Salman A, Vasuki V. The early history of glaucoma: The glaucous eye (800 BC to 1050 AD). Clin Ophthalmol. 2015;9:207–15.
2. Realini T. A history of glaucoma. Optom Vis Sci. 2011;88(1):36–8.
3. Leffler CT, Fan KW. The early history of glaucoma in East Asia. In: Leffler CT, Schwartz SG, editors. The History of Glaucoma. Ostend: Wayenborgh Publishing; 2020: 121–36.
4. Duke-Elder S. System of Ophthalmology. Vol XI: Diseases of the Lens and Vitreous; Glaucoma and Hypotony. London: Henry Kimpton; 1969.
5. Musa I, Bansal S, Kaleem MA. Barriers to care in the treatment of glaucoma: Socioeconomic elements that impact the diagnosis, treatment, and outcomes in glaucoma patients. Curr Ophthalmol Rep. 2022;10(3):85–90.
6. Shields MB. Normal-tension glaucoma: Is it different from primary open-angle glaucoma? Curr Opin Ophthalmol. 2008;19(2):85–8.
7. Fingeret M, Lewis TL. Primary Care of the Glaucomas. 2nd ed. New York: McGraw-Hill Medical; 2010.
8. Coleman AL, Miglior S. Risk factors for glaucoma onset and progression. Surv Ophthalmol. 2008;53(6 Suppl):S3–10.
9. Tham YC, Li X, Wong TY, Quigley HA, Aung T, Cheng CY. Global prevalence of glaucoma and projections of glaucoma burden through 2040: A systematic review and meta-analysis. Ophthalmology. 2014;121(11):2081–90.
10. Ehrlich JR, Burke-Conte Z, Wittenborn JS, Saaddine J, Omura JD. Prevalence of glaucoma among US adults in 2022. JAMA Ophthalmol. 2024;142(11):1046–53.
11. Varma R, Lee PP, Goldberg I, Kotak S. An assessment of the health and economic burdens of glaucoma. Am J Ophthalmol. 2011;152(4):515–22.
12. Centers for Disease Control and Prevention. Current Glaucoma Programs | Vision and Eye Health [Internet]. 2023 [cited 2025 Apr 16]. Available from: https://www.cdc.gov/vision-health/php/glaucoma-programs/index.html
13. Guedes RAP. Glaucoma, collective health and social impact. Rev Bras Oftalmol. 2021;80:5–7.
14. Gazzard G, Konstantakopoulou E, Garway-Heath D, Garg A, Vickerstaff V, Hunter R, et al. Selective laser trabeculoplasty versus eye drops for first-line treatment of ocular hypertension and glaucoma (LiGHT): A multicentre randomised controlled trial. Lancet. 2019;393(10180):1505–16.
15. Weinreb RN, Aung T, Medeiros FA. The pathophysiology and treatment of glaucoma: A review. JAMA. 2014;311(18):1901–11.

16. Medeiros FA, Zangwill LM, Bowd C, Mansouri K, Weinreb RN. The structure and function relationship in glaucoma: Implications for detection of progression and measurement of rates of change. Invest Ophthalmol Vis Sci. 2012;53(11):6939–46.

17. Flammer J, Mozaffarieh M. What is the present pathogenetic concept of glaucomatous optic neuropathy? Surv Ophthalmol. 2007;52(Suppl 2):S162–73.

18. Siesky BA, Harris A, Amireskandari A, Marek B. Glaucoma and ocular blood flow: An anatomical perspective. Expert Rev Ophthalmol. 2012;7(4):325–40.

19. Harris A, Jonescu-Cuypers CP. The impact of glaucoma medication on parameters of ocular perfusion. Curr Opin Ophthalmol. 2001 Apr 1;12(2):131–7.

20. Flammer J, Konieczka K. Retinal venous pressure: The role of endothelin. EPMA J. 2015;6:21.

21. Sigal IA, Yang H, Roberts MD, Burgoyne CF, Downs JC. IOP-induced lamina cribrosa displacement and scleral canal expansion: An analysis of factor interactions using parameterized eye-specific models. Invest Ophthalmol Vis Sci. 2011;52(3):1896–907.

22. Jonas JB, Berenshtein E, Holbach L. Anatomic relationship between lamina cribrosa, intraocular space, and cerebrospinal fluid space. Invest Ophthalmol Vis Sci. 2003;44(12):5189–95.

23. Stuntz M, Agarwal A, Christensen G, Nguyen QD. Normal histology of the uvea. In: The Uveitis Atlas. 1st ed. New York: Springer; 2020:3–6.

24. Kiel JW, Hollingsworth M, Rao R, Chen M, Reitsamer HA. Ciliary blood flow and aqueous humor production. Prog Retin Eye Res. 2011;30(1):1–17.

25. Goel M, Picciani RG, Lee RK, Bhattacharya SK. Aqueous humor dynamics: A review. Open Ophthalmol J. 2010;4:52–9.

26. Lam K, Lawlor M. Anatomy of the aqueous outflow drainage pathways. In: Minimally Invasive Glaucoma Surgery. Cham: Springer; 2021:11–19.

27. Yu DY, Cringle SJ, Balaratnasingam C, Morgan WH, Paula KY, Su EN. Retinal ganglion cells: Energetics, compartmentation, axonal transport, cytoskeletons and vulnerability. Prog Retin Eye Res. 2013;36:217–46.

28. Helvie R. Neural substrates of vision. In: Vision Rehabilitation: Multidisciplinary Care of the Patient Following Brain Injury. Boca Raton: CRC Press/Taylor & Francis; 2011.

29. Sambhara D, Aref AA. Glaucoma management: Relative value and place in therapy of available drug treatments. Ther Adv Chronic Dis. 2014;5(1):30–43.

30. Li F, Wang Z, Qu G, Song D, Yuan Y, Xu Y, et al. Automatic differentiation of glaucoma visual field from non-glaucoma visual field using deep convolutional neural network. BMC Med Imaging. 2018;18(1):35.

31. Stamer WD, Read AT, Sumida GM, Ethier CR. Sphingosine-1-phosphate effects on the inner wall of Schlemm's canal and outflow facility in perfused human eyes. Exp Eye Res. 2009;89(6):980–8.

32. Konstas AG, Quaranta L, Mikropoulos DG, Nasr MB, Russo A, Jaffee HA, et al. Twenty-four hour efficacy with preservative free tafluprost compared with latanoprost in patients with primary open angle glaucoma or ocular hypertension. Br J Ophthalmol. 2013;97(12):1510–5.

33. Newman-Casey PA, Blachley T, Lee PP, Heisler M, Farris KB, Stein JD. Patterns of glaucoma medication adherence over four years of follow-up. Ophthalmology. 2015;122(10):2010–21.

34. Robin AL, Novack GD, Covert DW, Crockett RS, Marcic TS. Adherence in glaucoma: Objective measurements of once-daily and adjunctive medication use. Am J Ophthalmol. 2007;144(4):533–40.

35. Okeke CO, Quigley HA, Jampel HD, Ying GS, Plyler RJ, Jiang Y, et al. Adherence with topical glaucoma medication monitored electronically: The Travatan Dosing Aid study. Ophthalmology. 2009;116(2):191–9.

36. Friedman DS, Hahn SR, Gelb L, Tan J, Shah SN, Kim EE, et al. Doctor-patient communication, health-related beliefs, and adherence in glaucoma: Results from the glaucoma adherence and persistency study. Ophthalmology. 2008;115(8):1320–7.

37. Campbell JH, Schwartz GF, LaBounty B, Kowalski JW, Patel VD. Patient adherence and persistence with topical ocular hypotensive therapy in real-world practice: A comparison of bimatoprost 0.01% and travoprost Z 0.004% ophthalmic solutions. Clin Ophthalmol. 2014;927–35.

38. Jayawant SS, Bhosle MJ, Anderson RT, Balkrishnan R. Depressive symptomatology, medication persistence, and associated healthcare costs in older adults with glaucoma. J Glaucoma. 2007;16(6):513–20.

39. Reardon G, Kotak S, Schwartz GF. Objective assessment of compliance and persistence among patients treated for glaucoma and ocular hypertension: A systematic review. Patient Prefer Adherence. 2011;5:441–63.

40. Stein JD, Shekhawat N, Talwar N, Balkrishnan R. Impact of the introduction of generic latanoprost on glaucoma medication adherence. Ophthalmology. 2015;122(4):738–47.

41. Hennessy AL, Katz J, Covert D, Protzko C, Robin AL. Videotaped evaluation of eyedrop instillation in glaucoma patients with visual impairment or moderate to severe visual field loss. Ophthalmology. 2010;117(12):2345–52.

42. Schlenker MB, Trope GE, Buys YM. Comparison of United States and Canadian glaucoma medication costs and price change from 2006 to 2013. J Ophthalmol. 2015;2015:547960.

43. Friedman DS, Okeke CO, Jampel HD, Ying GS, Plyler RJ, Jiang Y, et al. Risk factors for poor adherence to eyedrops in electronically monitored patients with glaucoma. Ophthalmology. 2009;116(6):1097–105.

44. Sleath B, Blalock SJ, Carpenter DM, Sayner R, Muir KW, Slota C, et al. Ophthalmologist–patient communication, self-efficacy, and glaucoma medication adherence. Ophthalmology. 2015;122(4):748–54.

45. Boland MV, Chang DS, Frazier T, Plyler R, Jefferys JL, Friedman DS. Automated telecommunication-based reminders and adherence with once-daily glaucoma medication dosing: The automated dosing reminder study. JAMA Ophthalmol. 2014;132(7):845–50.

46. Muir KW, Ventura A, Stinnett SS, Enfiedjian A, Allingham RR, Lee PP. The influence of health literacy level on an educational intervention to improve glaucoma medication adherence. Patient Educ Couns. 2012;87(2):160–4.

47. Fluorouracil Filtering Surgery Study Group. Five-year follow-up of the Fluorouracil Filtering Surgery Study. Am J Ophthalmol. 1996;121(4):349–66.

48. Gedde SJ, Schiffman JC, Feuer WJ, Herndon LW, Brandt JD, Budenz DL, et al. Treatment outcomes in the Tube versus Trabeculectomy (TVT) study after five years of follow-up. Am J Ophthalmol. 2012;153(5):789–803.

49. Rulli E, Biagioli E, Riva I, Gambirasio G, De Simone I, Floriani I, et al. Efficacy and safety of trabeculectomy vs nonpenetrating surgical procedures: A systematic review and meta-analysis. JAMA Ophthalmol. 2013;131(12):1573–82.

50. Samuelson TW, Katz LJ, Wells JM, Duh YJ, Giamporcaro JE; US iStent Study Group. Randomized evaluation of the trabecular micro-bypass stent with phacoemulsification in patients with glaucoma and cataract. Ophthalmology. 2011;118(3):459–67.

51. Mansouri K, Guidotti J, Rao HL, Ouabas A, D'Alessandro E, Roy S, et al. Prospective evaluation of standalone XEN Gel implant and combined phacoemulsification-XEN Gel implant surgery: 1-year results. J Glaucoma. 2018;27(2):140–7.

52. Aquino MCD, Barton K, Tan AMW, Sng C, Li X, Loon SC, et al. Micropulse versus continuous wave transscleral diode cyclophotocoagulation in refractory glaucoma: A randomized exploratory study. Clin Exp Ophthalmol. 2015;43(1):40–6.

53. Rao HL, Pradhan ZS, Suh MH, Moghimi S, Mansouri K, Weinreb RN. Optical coherence tomography angiography in glaucoma. J Glaucoma. 2020;29(4):312–21.

54. Ting DSW, Cheung CY, Lim G, Tan GSW, Quang ND, Gan A, et al. Development and validation of a deep learning system for diabetic retinopathy and related eye diseases using retinal images from multiethnic populations with diabetes. JAMA. 2017;318(22):2211–23.

55. Cheng L, Sapieha P, Kittlerova P, Hauswirth WW, Di Polo A. TrkB gene transfer protects retinal ganglion cells from axotomy-induced death in vivo. J Neurosci. 2002;22(10):3977–86.

56. Venugopalan P, Wang Y, Nguyen T, Huang A, Muller KJ, Goldberg JL. Transplanted neurons integrate into adult retinas and respond to light. Nat Commun. 2016;7(1):10472.

57. Khawaja AP, Cooke Bailey JN, Wareham NJ, Scott RA, Simcoe M, Igo RP Jr, et al. Genome-wide analyses identify 68 new loci associated with intraocular pressure and improve risk prediction for primary open-angle glaucoma. Nat Genet. 2018;50(6):778–82.

58. Christopher M, Belghith A, Bowd C, Proudfoot JA, Goldbaum MH, Weinreb RN, et al. Performance of deep learning architectures and transfer learning for detecting glaucomatous optic neuropathy in fundus photographs. Sci Rep. 2018;8(1):16685.

59. Mendicino ME, Lynch MG, Drack A, Beck AD, Harbin T, Pollard Z, et al. Long-term surgical and visual outcomes in primary congenital glaucoma: 360 trabeculotomy versus goniotomy. J AAPOS. 2000;4(4):205–10.

60. Siddique SS, Suelves AM, Baheti U, Foster CS. Glaucoma and uveitis. Surv Ophthalmol. 2013;58(1):1–10.

61. Liu S, Lin Y, Liu X. Meta-analysis of association of obstructive sleep apnea with glaucoma. J Glaucoma. 2016;25(1):1–7.
62. Gyasi ME, Amoaku WMK, Debrah OA, Awini EA, Abugri P. Outcome of trabeculectomies without adjunctive antimetabolites. Ghana Med J. 2006; 40(2):39–43.
63. Bastawrous A, Rono HK, Livingstone IA, Weiss HA, Jordan S, Kuper H, et al. Development and validation of a smartphone-based visual acuity test (peek acuity) for clinical practice and community-based fieldwork. JAMA Ophthalmol. 2015;133(8):930 7.
64. Resnikoff S, Lansingh VC, Washburn L, Felch W, Gauthier TM, Taylor HR, et al. Estimated number of ophthalmologists worldwide (International Council of Ophthalmology update): Will we meet the needs? Br J Ophthalmol. 2020;104(4):588–92.
65. Thomas SM, Jeyaraman M, Hodge WG, Hutnik C, Costella J, Malvankar-Mehta MS. The effectiveness of teleglaucoma versus in-patient examination for glaucoma screening: A systematic review and meta-analysis. PLoS One. 2014;9(12):e113779.
66. Hu GY, Prasad J, Chen DK, Alcantara-Castillo JC, Patel VN, Al-Aswad LA. Home monitoring of glaucoma using a home tonometer and a novel virtual reality visual field device: Acceptability and feasibility. Ophthalmol Glaucoma. 2023;6(2):121–8.
67. Ramke J, Petkovic J, Welch V, Blignault I, Gilbert C, Blanchet K, et al. Interventions to improve access to cataract surgical services and their impact on equity in low- and middle-income countries. Cochrane Database Syst Rev. 2017;(11):CD011307.
68. Greenfield DS, Siatkowski RM, Glaser JS, Schatz NJ, Parrish RK 2nd. The cupped disc: Who needs neuroimaging? Ophthalmology. 1998;105(10):1866–74.
69. Bae SH, Kang SH, Feng CS, Park J, Jeong JH, Yi K. Influence of myopia on size of optic nerve head and retinal nerve fiber layer thickness measured by spectral domain optical coherence tomography. Korean J Ophthalmol. 2016;30(5):335.
70. Peng PH, Nguyen H, Lin HS, Nguyen N, Lin S. Long-term outcomes of laser iridotomy in Vietnamese patients with primary angle closure. Br J Ophthalmol. 2011;95(9):1207–11.
71. Ritch R, Chang BM, Liebmann JM. Angle closure in younger patients. Ophthalmology. 2003;110(10):1880–9.
72. Grover DS, Godfrey DG, Smith O, Feuer WJ, de Oca IM, Fellman RL. Gonioscopy-assisted transluminal trabeculotomy, ab interno trabeculotomy: Technique report and preliminary results. Ophthalmology. 2014;121(4):855–61.
73. Grover DS, Smith O, Fellman RL, Godfrey DG, Gupta A, de Oca IM, et al. Gonioscopy-assisted transluminal trabeculotomy: An ab interno circumferential trabeculotomy: 24 months follow-up. J Glaucoma. 2018;27(5):393–401.
74. Benson SE, Mandal K, Bunce CV, Fraser SG. Is post-trabeculectomy hypotony a risk factor for subsequent failure? A case control study. BMC Ophthalmol. 2005;5:1–5.

75. Leske MC, Heijl A, Hyman L, Bengtsson B, Dong L, Yang Z, et al. Predictors of long-term progression in the early manifest glaucoma trial. Ophthalmology. 2007;114(11):1965–72.

76. Glen FC, Crabb DP. Living with glaucoma: A qualitative study of functional implications and patients' coping behaviours. BMC Ophthalmol. 2015;15:128.

77. Memon MS, Shaikh SA, Shaikh AR, Fahim MF, Mumtaz SN, Ahmed N. An assessment of knowledge, attitude and practices (KAP) towards diabetes and diabetic retinopathy in a suburban town of Karachi. Pak J Med Sci. 2015;31(1):183–8.

78. Wang SY, Singh K, Lin SC. Prevalence and predictors of depression among participants with glaucoma in a nationally representative population sample. Am J Ophthalmol. 2012;154(3):436–44.

INDEX

Page numbers in *italics* indicate figures; page numbers in **bold** indicate tables.

For Product Safety Concerns and Information please contact our EU
representative GPSR@taylorandfrancis.com
Taylor & Francis Verlag GmbH, Kaufingerstraße 24, 80331 München, Germany

www.ingramcontent.com/pod-product-compliance
Lightning Source LLC
Chambersburg PA
CBHW070724220326
41598CB00024BA/3284